EPILEPSY
199
ANSWERS

ANDREW N. WILNER, MD, FACP, FAAN

EPILEPSY 199 ANSWERS

A DOCTOR RESPONDS TO HIS PATIENTS' QUESTIONS

THIRD EDITION

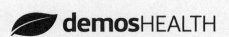 demosHEALTH

Library of Congress Cataloging-in-Publication Data
Wilner, Andrew N.
  Epilepsy : 199 answers : a doctor responds to his patients' questions / Andrew N. Wilner. – 3rd ed.
    p. cm.
  ISBN-13: 978-1-932603-35-4 (pbk. : alk. paper)
  ISBN-10: 1-932603-35-2 (pbk. : alk. paper)
  1. Epilepsy--Popular Works. 2. Epilepsy--Miscellanea. I. Title.
  RC372.W55 2008
  616.8'53--dc22

                    2007047850

Medicine is an ever-changing science undergoing continual development. Research and clinical experience are continually expanding our knowledge, in particular our knowledge of proper treatment and drug therapy. The authors, editors, and publisher have made every effort to ensure that all information in this book is in accordance with the state of knowledge at the time of production of the book.

Nevertheless, this does not imply or express any guarantee or responsibility on the part of the authors, editors, or publisher with respect to any dosage instructions and forms of application stated in the book. Every reader should examine carefully the package inserts accompanying each drug and check with a physician or specialist whether the dosage schedules mentioned therein or the contraindications stated by the manufacturer differ from the statements made in this book. Such examination is particularly important with drugs that are either rarely used or have been newly released on the market. Every dosage schedule or every form of application used is entirely at the reader's own risk and responsibility. The editors and publisher welcome any reader to report to the publisher any discrepancies or inaccuracies noticed.

SPECIAL DISCOUNTS ON BULK QUANTITIES of Demos Medical Publishing books are available to corporations, professional associations, pharmaceutical companies, health care organizations, and other qualifying groups. For details, please contact:

        Special Sales Department
        Demos Medical Publishing
        386 Park Avenue South, Suite 301
        New York, NY 10016
        Phone: 800–532–8663 or 212–683–0072
        Fax: 212–683–0118
        E-mail: orderdept@demosmedpub.com

Made in the United States of America
07 08 09 10 5 4 3 2 1

TO
My Family

ACKNOWLEDGMENTS

I WOULD LIKE TO EXPRESS GRATITUDE to my teachers at the Montreal Neurological Institute, in particular Drs. Fred Andermann, Peter Gloor, and Felipe Quesney, for introducing me to the wonderful mysteries of epilepsy and clinical neurophysiology. Both Drs. Gloor and Quesney are now deceased, but I hope their legacy of fine teaching lives on at least in some small way in this new edition of *Epilepsy: 199 Answers*.

The lessons I have learned come from my experience in treating more than 1,000 people with epilepsy. Over the years, I have tried my best to answer their questions as they have struggled with mine. The "199 Answers" of this book evolved from our many discussions. Any value in this book derives from our work together to control their seizures.

The keen academic atmosphere provided by my partners and colleagues at the Carolinas Epilepsy Center and the staff of Carolina Neurological Clinic, P.A., provided a supportive atmosphere for the writing of the first edition of *Epilepsy: 199 Answers*, which was published more than a decade ago. I wrote the second edition after working as an Associate Clinical Professor of Neurology at Brown University. This third edition finds me immersed in the field of medical journalism, communicating advances in neurology through news stories written both for physician and lay audiences, creating continuing medical education programs for physicians, as well as writing for the American Epilepsy Society, American Academy of Neurology, Epilepsy Foundation, and other organizations focused on improving the lives of people with epilepsy and other neurological disorders. As a medical journalist, I regularly attend many medical conferences and interview hundreds of researchers. I continue to see patients with epilepsy and other medical disorders as a volunteer in medical clinics in underserved areas.

The American Epilepsy Society, Epilepsy Foundation, International Bureau for Epilepsy, and International League Against Epilepsy provided much valuable resource material. In addition, this book has benefited from discussions with many colleagues who provided valuable insight and information that I have incorporated into the text. While it would be impossible to acknowledge everyone who has contributed, I would like to thank those who provided specific information or reviewed parts of the manuscript, including Bassel Abou-Khalil, MD, Jorge Asconape, MD, Orly Avitzur, MD, Paul Cooper, DM, FRCP, Sandra Cushner-Weinstein, RPT, LCSW-C, David Dunn, MD, Jen Frank, Matthew Frank, MD, Joseph Friedman, MD, Patricia Gibson, MSSW, Barry Gidal, PharmD, Natasha Green, Robert Gross, MD, Christina Gurnett, MD, PhD, Cynthia Harden, MD, Amy Kaloides, Hoon-Chul Kang, MD, PhD, Eric Kossoff, MD, Kimford Meador, MD, Roger Porter, MD, Caitlin Reilly Smith, MPH, Michael Smith, MD, Susan Cole Stone, George Trksak, PhD, and Ponpimon Vongchedkuan.

Any errors are my own responsibility. I welcome corrections and updates for the next edition.

Although I have endeavored to include as much important information for people with epilepsy as is possible to fit in this little book, I make no claim that this book is "complete." Given the rapid "information explosion" of modern times, such a book would be too heavy to carry around and could never be finished!

I urge interested readers to consult with their health care providers, friends, and family for additional resources, and of course, to seek out the references provided in the Appendices.

I also thank my agent and publisher for their kind and persistent assistance.

And last, but not least, I would like to thank the many thousands of readers who warmly received the first two editions of *Epilepsy: 199 Answers*, giving impetus to the creation of this third edition.

CONTENTS

2. Why So Many Tests?   11

3. At the Doctor's Office   17

8. Can I Drive?   73

9. Seizures and Work   79

10. Women and Epilepsy   89

13. First Aid and Safety Tips   113

14. Clinical Research: Should I Participate in a Drug Trial?   121

15. Who Else Can Help?   131

Foreword

A S A BUSY EPILEPSY specialist and researcher, I am always trying to find better ways to ensure that my patients are getting the best possible information about their condition. In an ideal world, my first visit would be scheduled to last several hours, because there is so much important information that needs to be exchanged. Unfortunately, one single hour is all I can usually spend. Even if I had the necessary time to tell my patients everything they need to know, many would get home and remember several more questions they didn't have time to ask, or realize that they should have written everything down, because they are unable to recall exactly what the doctor said. That is why this book is so valuable. If this book is available and read before the doctor's visit, it will enable a patient or family member to get the most out of the time that they have with their physician. By reading this book, they are able to find answers to many questions in advance, and they will be better prepared to understand what the doctor is discussing. In addition, if each patient came to their first visit with a completed health record (see Appendix A), it would save valuable time the doctor would otherwise spend obtaining this information. In fact, this form is so complete, it could easily result in the doctor having access to information he or she might not have thought to inquire about and could improve diagnosis and treatment selection.

This book is also valuable after the first doctor's visit, and at any time thereafter. Some issues may not have arisen during the doctor's visit, such as dealing with employment issues, deciding when it may be time to move on to epilepsy surgery, or thinking about becoming involved in a clinical trial. In other areas, the book also discusses more in-depth answers than the treating physician often provides. For example, the doctor may tell you that you are not eligible to drive, but may not have time to go into all the issues that are dealt with in the book.

The resource guide, alone, makes the book well worth having. It is difficult to get access to important information such as brand and generic drug names, listings of pharmaceutical companies that manufacture antiepileptic drugs, comprehensive epilepsy centers, driving laws by state, and important internet resources.

This new edition also provides cutting edge updates, including information on new drugs and technology that was not available at the time of the writing of the previous edition. Dr. Wilner has included information about new devices, such as the Deep Brain Stimulator and the Responsive Neurostimulator, that are currently undergoing clinical trials.

A great advantage of this book is that Dr. Wilner is not only an experienced epilepsy physician; he is also an accomplished communicator. The book is written in a straightforward, honest, and simple to understand style. I would be happy to have this book in the hands of all my patients.

Jacqueline A. French, MD
Professor
New York University School of Medicine
New York University Comprehensive Epilepsy Center

Introduction

WHEN YOU READ *Epilepsy: 199 Answers*, you will learn
more about the large group of diseases known as epilepsy.
You will understand your doctor's language and ask better questions. If you fill in the medical history section, keep your calendar, and carry this book when you visit your doctor, it will help
you receive optimal care.

I wrote this book on the premise that accurate and compre-
hensible medical information can empower people with epilepsy
to combat their disease.

To complete the first chapter, "What Is Epilepsy?," demanded
that I harness all my training and experience. Epilepsy is something different for each one of my patients. For some, it is a rare
convulsion, imposing the inconvenience of daily antiepileptic
medication and a yearly visit to my office. For others, frequent
seizures are part of a devastating constellation of brain injury,
mental impairment, and social problems. These people come to
my office accompanied by concerned and often exhausted caregiv-
ers, desperately searching for a solution to multiple disabilities
of which epilepsy is merely one. In writing this book, I have tried
to address the needs of all people with epilepsy, whether their
epilepsy is mild or severe.

The positive feedback from readers of the first two editions
of *Epilepsy: 199 Answers* encouraged me to write an updated
and significantly enlarged third edition. Although the principles

of epilepsy management have not changed, our sophistication regarding antiepileptic drugs, brain stimulation, diet therapy, neuroimaging, and surgical treatment has dramatically improved since *Epilepsy: 199 Answers* was first published in 1996. It is my hope that anyone with epilepsy, a family member, or health care worker who is searching for information and encouragement regarding epilepsy will find their efforts rewarded within the pages of this book. While the number of chapters remains at sixteen, nearly all of them have increased in size to accommodate the new information available. Four new appendices have been added, including a home safety checklist, epilepsy first aid, an epilepsy "action plan" for the workplace, and other epilepsy resources. The glossary of terms has nearly doubled in size. Both the text and resource sections have been completely rewritten to reflect the state of the art of epilepsy treatment in 2008.

Since the publication of the first edition of *Epilepsy: 199 Answers*, the US Food and Drug Administration (FDA) has approved five new antiepileptic drugs; levetiracetam (Keppra®), oxcarbazepine (Trileptal®), pregabalin (Lyrica®), tiagabine (Gabitril®), and zonisamide (Zonegran®). Although none of these drugs is a miracle cure, many patients have benefited with fewer seizures or decreased side effects. The effects of inflation may also be seen. In 1996, I addressed the problem of antiepileptic drugs costing "one or two dollars" a pill. For this edition, I had to change it to "three or four dollars."

More than 20 new antiepileptic drugs are in development, and some or all of these may prove beneficial for people with epilepsy in the near future. Another new treatment, the vagus nerve stimulator, received FDA approval in 1997 and has found increasing acceptance in the epilepsy community. More than 40,000 vagus nerve stimulators have been implanted worldwide for people with intractable epilepsy. The next generation of vagus nerve stimulators, which are 40% smaller, recently received FDA approval (July 2007). In addition, a responsive brain stimulator, designed to be implanted in the brain, detects seizures and stops them with a small electric pulse, has begun clinical trials in select patients with intractable epilepsy.

The impressive growth in the number of comprehensive epilepsy centers is testimony to the increased recognition of the importance of epilepsy as a treatable disorder. The number of comprehensive epilepsy centers has more than doubled since the publication of the second edition of *Epilepsy: 199 Answers*, from 52 in 2003 to 118 in 2007. In addition, member organizations of the International Bureau for Epilepsy have grown from 58 in 2003 to 87 in 2007, exemplifying an increase in awareness of epilepsy and support for people with epilepsy worldwide.

Since 1996 the use of magnetic resonance imaging has become much more widespread, leading to more precise diagnoses of the cause of epilepsy in many patients. In particular, mesial temporal sclerosis and neuronal migration disorders are recognized far more frequently. This advance in diagnostic precision has improved patient care. Epilepsy due to mesial temporal sclerosis can often be cured by epilepsy surgery, and neuronal migration disorders may have important genetic implications.

Our understanding of the genetic basis of epilepsy continues to grow. More than 200 genes have been identified that are responsible for epilepsy or neurological syndromes associated with epilepsy. A large research effort is directed to creating new drugs that target the abnormal products of these genes. Commercial gene testing is now becoming available. There is every reason to believe that new and more effective approaches to the treatment of epilepsy will be available in the near future.

The resurgence of interest in diet therapy has led to many more studies of the ketogenic diet and now the modified Atkins diet as treatments for refractory seizures. Many patients, especially children, benefit from these special diets, and they provide an alternative or supplement to traditional antiepileptic medication therapy.

The North American Pregnancy Registry, established in 1996, has enrolled over 5,600 women who are taking antiepileptic drugs and begun to publish data regarding the risk of birth defects and developmental impairment from various antiepileptic drugs. (This enrollment has more than doubled since the last edition.) A European Pregnancy Registry and other patient registries have also commenced work on this problem. In the years to come, the information gathered by these registries will help guide antiepileptic drug selection for women of childbearing age.

In terms of the place of epilepsy in our society, it is my impression that there is a greater understanding among lay people about the nature of epilepsy. Although the stigma of epilepsy has not disappeared, it seems that with continued public education this problem will continue to diminish. One piece of evidence to support this feeling is that driving restrictions for people with controlled seizures have eased in several states, enhancing the chances that someone with epilepsy will be able to obtain a driver's license.

Recognition by health care professionals of the high prevalence of mental health issues such as depression and anxiety in people with epilepsy and the need to address them has increased over the last decade. The detrimental effects of these comorbidities on quality of life have become apparent, leading to more research and treatment of psychiatric and behavioral issues.

Another interesting change since 1996 is our evolving concept of who constitutes the "elderly." While the conventional definition of elderly is older than age 65 years, it is not rare to see active septuagenarians and older people in doctors' offices, on golf courses, and in the workplace. When I first wrote the chapter "Epilepsy and the Elderly" 12 years ago, the elderly patient I chose for the case study was a mere 66 years old, a "spring chicken" by today's standards! Research into the special considerations of diagnosing and managing epilepsy in the elderly is increasing and is reflected in this updated chapter.

Since the first publication of *Epilepsy: 199 Answers*, epilepsy resources have become much more widely available on the internet. For this edition, I have included the most useful resources that I could find. Other valuable internet resources may exist and new ones are sure to crop up by the time this book is published. As with any information resource, be sure to examine the website closely to insure that the information is of high quality and applies to you.

The clinical scenarios in this book are based on patients in my own practice. To insure patient privacy, none of the names used in the case histories is real. For the same reason, I have changed some details or combined the stories of two patients into one. But these case studies are not imagined or hypothetical; they illustrate the real problems faced by people with epilepsy.

When referring to "your doctor," I have consistently used the pronoun *he* rather than the awkward *he/she*. Historically, neurologists have been male. For example, 90% of senior members of the American Academy of Neurology are men. However, more and more women have taken an interest in neurology. Women neurologists now comprise 25% of the active membership of the American Academy of Neurology, and 48% of the student membership are women. (If your neurologist is a woman, feel free to add a preceding "s" to "he.")

Epilepsy: 199 Answers is a valuable tool to help you understand and cope with seizures. Use the resource section that lists the many organizations devoted to helping people with epilepsy. The Epilepsy Foundation, American Epilepsy Society, International Bureau for Epilepsy, International League Against Epilepsy, and many other organizations can provide assistance. Seek out a Comprehensive Epilepsy Center if you need one. Relevant telephone numbers, addresses, and websites are listed in the back of the book. Do not hesitate to use them. I have tried to make the reference section of this book as complete as possible, and all references have been updated for this new edition. Suggestions for additional reading are in the bibliography, including patient information books, books relating the personal experiences of people with epilepsy, and information books for children with epilepsy.

A glance at the time line in the front of this book reveals that most of the significant advances in understanding epilepsy have occurred in the last hundred years, many in just the last decade. In the twenty-first century, there are more proven treatments for epilepsy than ever before. Modern medicine really can help people with epilepsy! Based on my experience attending many medical conferences and interviewing epilepsy researchers, it is my prediction that the next decade will show even more dramatic progress. Work with your doctor and health care team and reap the benefits of modern medicine. Good luck in taking control of your epilepsy!

Over the years, it has been gratifying to meet people who have benefited from reading my book. One of my favorite experiences occurred at a medical conference with a neurologist from Eastern Europe. She was very pleased to meet me because I had the same name as *the* Dr. Wilner who wrote *Epilepsy: 199 Answers*, which had helped many of her patients! I hope this third edition of *Epilepsy: 199 Answers* continues to be a source of sound information and hope for people with epilepsy.

Time Line

400 BC	Hippocrates writes first book on epilepsy, *On the Sacred Disease*
1543	Andreas Vesalius, founder of modern anatomy, publishes *De Humani Corporis Fabrica*
1754	Pedro de Horta writes the first epilepsy textbook in the Western Hemisphere
1857	Charles Locock finds bromide effective for seizure control
1873	Hughlings Jackson correctly defines epilepsy as "the name for occasional, sudden, excessive, rapid, and local discharges of grey matter"
1886	First successful resective surgery for partial seizures by Victor Horsley
1895	Discovery of x-rays by Konrad Roentgen
1912	Phenobarbital introduced
1921	R. M. Wilder introduces the ketogenic diet as treatment for epilepsy
1929	Hans Berger invents the electroencephalogram
1935	Gibbs, Davis, and Lennox publish the first description of spike and wave discharge from patients with petit mal seizures
1937	Merritt and Putnam demonstrate the antiepileptic action of phenytoin (Dilantin®)
1938	Herbert Jasper organizes a laboratory of electroencephalography at the Montreal Neurological Institute and collaborates with Wilder Penfield, the renowned epilepsy neurosurgeon

1954	Establishment of the American Epilepsy Society, a professional group dedicated to supporting individuals affected by epilepsy through research, education, and advocacy
1968	Establishment of the Epilepsy Foundation, a national voluntary health organization devoted to helping people with epilepsy
1972	Early images of first computed axial tomography (CAT or CT) scanner
1973	Passage of antidiscriminatory Rehabilitation Act
1974	Carbamazepine (Tegretol®) introduced in United States
1975	First comprehensive epilepsy centers established in United States
1978	Valproic acid (Depakene®) introduced in United States
1980	Positron emission tomography (PET) scan identifies epileptic patterns of local cerebral metabolism
1981	Magnetic resonance imaging (MRI) introduced into clinical medicine
1988	First vagus nerve stimulator implanted in human being
1990	Passage of the Americans with Disabilities Act
1993	Felbamate (Felbatol®) receives FDA approval for add-on and monotherapy
1994	Gabapentin (Neurontin®) and lamotrigine (Lamictal®) receive FDA approval
1996	Fosphenytoin (Cerebyx®) and topiramate (Topamax®) receive FDA approval
1997	Tiagabine (Gabitril®) and vagus nerve stimulator receive FDA approval
1999	Levetiracetam (Keppra®) receives FDA approval
2000	Oxcarbazepine (Trileptal®) and zonisamide (Zonegran®) receive FDA approval
2005	Pregabalin (Lyrica®) receives FDA approval

EPILEPSY
199
ANSWERS

WHAT IS EPILEPSY?

> **B**rian handed me his seizure calendar and piled five medication bottles on my desk. I picked up his thick chart, asked him how things were going and started to write my office note. As I recorded his seizure frequency and drug dosages, a loud wailing sound startled me. I looked up and saw Brian's right arm and leg slowly extend and his whole body stiffen. Then the frightening sound stopped. His eyes closed, and he smacked his lips for fifteen seconds. Then his body relaxed, and he slumped in the chair.
>
> After the seizure, Brian was sleepy and confused. I made sure he didn't fall off the chair or wander out of the room. He couldn't answer any questions for about ten minutes. When he became more alert, I told Brian he'd had a seizure.

1. What is epilepsy?

Epilepsy is a group of brain disorders characterized by recurrent seizures that occurs in 0.5 to 1% of the world's population. There are approximately 2.7 million Americans with epilepsy. Physicians diagnose 200,000 new cases of epilepsy each year. A variety of insults to the brain may result in epilepsy such as a birth defect, birth injury, bleeding in the brain, brain infection, brain tumor, head injury, or stroke. Some cases of epilepsy are inherited. Scientists have identified more than 200 abnormal genes associated with epilepsy. However, in approximately 50% of people with epilepsy, even after a thorough investigation, a cause cannot be found. When patients come to me with epilepsy, my job is to find and treat its cause and then prescribe treatment to diminish the severity and frequency of the seizures. The goal of epilepsy treatment is complete seizure control without side effects.

2. What is a seizure?

A seizure is an abnormal electrical discharge of a group of neurons in the brain. Seizures can produce a variety of symptoms, depending on the location of the seizure focus and the spread of the abnormal electrical activity through the brain. Some of these symptoms may be very strange and unusual. Here are some examples from patients in my practice.

After a small stroke, my partner's elderly mother, Susan, experiences minor seizures, which consist only of a tingling in her right forefinger. Karen has a "funny feeling in my stomach," then becomes confused. Jim has a "vague feeling that I'm losing touch with reality." On one occasion, he saw the refrigerator "singing a melody." Alan typically has a feeling that "whatever I am thinking about has happened before," then blacks out. Mary has a feeling that "something isn't right," and her head becomes "numb." She stares, wraps her arms around herself, and rolls up in a ball. Ron has a warning of a "tingling feeling in my mind" followed by loss of consciousness and a fall.

Many of my patients have convulsions, hard seizures during which they lose consciousness, become stiff, and jerk. Richard only has convulsions twice a year, but when he does, they can last for hours, a life-threatening condition called "status epilepticus" (Question #16). He comes by ambulance to the hospital for an admission to the intensive care unit where we stop the seizures with intravenous antiepileptic medications.

Experiencing or watching a seizure can be unsettling. It takes some getting used to.

3. What do I do about a first seizure?

Everyone with a first seizure requires a prompt thorough neurological evaluation in an attempt to determine the cause of the seizure. All treatment decisions stem from this first evaluation.

Brian's magnetic resonance imaging (MRI) scan revealed that part of his left frontal lobe had not developed properly when he was in the womb. This was the cause of his seizures. Another of my patients had a seizure while walking outside to pick up a newspaper. It began with an unpleasant odor. His computed axial tomography (CAT or CT) scan was normal, but the more sensitive MRI revealed a tiny tumor in his left temporal lobe, which we treated with radiation and surgery. A young woman had a seizure while working as a receptionist in a local hotel. Her MRI demonstrated evidence of multiple sclerosis, a relatively uncommon cause of seizures.

4. I've only had one seizure. Do I have epilepsy?

Epilepsy is a clinical condition defined by recurrent seizures. Technically, you do not have epilepsy if you have only had one seizure. From a practical standpoint, often sophisticated testing, such as electroencephalography (EEG) and brain imaging with a computed axial tomography (CAT or CT) or magnetic resonance imaging (MRI) scan can predict the likelihood of a second seizure and greatly influence whether you need antiepileptic medication.

Not all seizures are epilepsy. For example, withdrawal from alcohol or addicting drugs can stress the body and cause a seizure. If this circumstance is not repeated, the seizure will not recur. This type of provoked seizure is not classified as epilepsy.

5. At what age does epilepsy occur?

Epilepsy can begin at any age. It can occur immediately after birth or for the first time in old age. In fact, very young and very old people are more likely to develop epilepsy.

6. Is it contagious?

No.

7. Why me? Why do I have epilepsy?

In order to answer this question, you will probably need to see a neurologist who will ask you many questions and perform a detailed examination of your nervous system. You will have a brain scan, either a computed axial tomography (CAT or CT) or magnetic resonance imaging (MRI) scan, and a brain wave test (electroencephalograph).

In some cases, a treatable cause will be found, such as a brain tumor, which may be removed. In others, the cause will be attributed to a past head injury or brain infection. In many patients, no cause will be found. See Chapters 2 and 3 for more details.

8. How do I know if it is an epileptic seizure?

Not every spell is an epileptic seizure. Some people faint after donating blood, followed by jerking movements. Others collapse because of an abnormal heart rhythm. People with diabetes can become confused or unresponsive as a result of low blood sugar. Sometimes people pass out under severe emotional stress.

When I evaluate a patient for suspected epilepsy, I spend a lot of time trying to determine whether a particular spell was an epileptic seizure, another neurological or medical disorder, or a psychological problem. Short of recording the event on video and examining the brain waves, the best tool to solve this puzzle is an accurate and detailed account of what actually happened. It is very helpful if you can bring a witness when you visit your doctor. Video and electroencephalographic (Video/EEG) recording can be done at home or in the hospital in difficult to diagnose cases.

9. My doctor said I have a seizure disorder. Is that the same thing as epilepsy?

Most likely, yes. In the past, some physicians avoided using the word *epilepsy* in order not to upset patients who mistakenly believed epilepsy to be a mental illness. These misunderstandings are much less common now. My own approach is to inform patients of their diagnosis rather than beat around the bush. In this way, patients can educate themselves and their families and learn to cope with the reality of their illness.

10. My father had complications from cardiac bypass surgery and had his first seizure in the hospital. Does he have epilepsy?

Sometimes people have seizures due to a severe illness, such as pneumonia with kidney and liver problems, or following a difficult operation. In such circumstances, temporary brain dysfunction caused by the illness results in seizures. The seizures disappear when the illness improves. These seizures are not epilepsy.

11. What is the best diagnostic test for epilepsy?

There is no blood test or other definitive test for epilepsy. The diagnosis of epilepsy must be made by a physician who incorporates the history, physical and neurological examination, and test results into a diagnosis. The most useful test for the neurologist is the electroencephalograph (EEG), which amplifies a patient's brain waves and records them on paper or displays them on a video screen. In people with epilepsy, a typical pattern of "spikes" occurs during an epileptic seizure. In between seizures, spikes may not be present and the diagnosis can be more difficult. For this reason, multiple EEGs may be needed before a definite diagnosis of epilepsy is made.

Other tests, such as computed axial tomography (CAT or CT scan) and magnetic resonance imaging (MRI), provide a detailed picture of the brain. These scans can reveal birth defects, tumors, and other brain abnormalities that may cause epilepsy.

12. How will epilepsy affect my life?

As you can imagine from the previous case histories, epilepsy affects each person differently. For some people, epilepsy is a childhood condition they outgrow. For others, daily falls and frequent trips to the emergency room for cuts and bruises painfully remind them of the defect in their brain. Seizures restrict driving, social opportunities, ability to work and hurt self-esteem. Many people with epilepsy suffer comorbid psychiatric conditions, such as anxiety and depression, which may need to be treated as well.

Most patients' seizures can be controlled with antiepileptic medication. About half see their seizures disappear with the first medication they try. Others require multiple doctor visits to find the dosage and combination of medications that control their seizures without intolerable side effects. Many antiepileptic drugs are available to try (Chapters 4 and 5 and Appendix B).

A new research drug may be the answer for some patients (Chapter 14). Others will stop having seizures only when their seizure focus is surgically removed (Chapter 7). Diet therapy (Question #147) and the vagus nerve stimulator (Question #73) are additional options.

13. What can I do to control my seizures?

Become part of the health care team! The knowledge you gain from reading this book will give you the background to better understand your medical problem and therapeutic options. When you fill in the medical history section and seizure calendar in the back of this book, it will enable you to actively participate in your doctor's decisions about antiepileptic medications and other treatment.

Learn to effectively communicate with your doctor and his staff. They are there to help you. Bring all your medications to each doctor visit.

There are three simple things you can do to decrease the severity and frequency of your seizures.

○ Take your antiepileptic medication regularly. Linking the medication to another routine can help you to remember it. Many of my patients take their medications three times a day, once with each meal. If you take medication only twice a day, the first dose can be when you brush your teeth in the morning and the second when you prepare for bed. There are memory aids that can assist you. One of my patients has a watch that beeps when another dose is due. Another has a watch with a voice synthesizer to remind him. Use a pillbox if you need one. You can buy an inexpensive one at a pharmacy.

○ Get enough sleep! Rob only has seizures when he is sleep deprived. His seizures are severe and he ends up in the hospital. Once he was almost arrested because his behavior was so bizarre after a seizure; just because he didn't get a good night's sleep the day before!

○ Follow up regularly with your doctor so that you can work together. If you are having seizures, you need to adjust your antiepileptic medication dosage or switch to another medication. Make a new appointment each time you leave the office so that the doctor can evaluate your progress. Try not to miss appointments. Remember, your doctor can't help you if you don't show up!

14. What is intractable epilepsy?

Patients whose seizures recur despite intensive and regular treatment with antiepileptic medications have intractable, refractory, or uncontrolled epilepsy. These patients often resort to new research drugs (Chapter 14) or seizure surgery (Chapter 7) because their epilepsy is so difficult to control.

15. Can I die during a seizure?

The death rate for people with epilepsy is two to three times that of the general population. Death from a seizure is extremely rare, but it can occur. Seizures can cause accidents as well as irregular heart rhythms. See Chapter 13 for epilepsy first aid and tips on accident prevention.

In my practice of hundreds of patients with thousands of seizures, two people have died as a direct result of epilepsy. One drowned in a whirlpool at the YMCA (where he should not have gone alone). The other was found in bed, the cause of death unknown. This may have been a case of SUDEP (sudden unexpected [unexplained] death in epilepsy), a rare condition defined as a sudden, unexpected death in someone with epilepsy without an identifiable cause. SUDEP accounts for less than 25% of deaths in people with epilepsy. Heart and/or lung failure seem to be responsible. Because SUDEP is so rare and unpredictable, it is difficult to study. SUDEP is more common in young (ages 20 to 40) people with intractable epilepsy, epilepsy for ten years or more, and a seizure within the last year. Seizure control may decrease the risk of SUDEP.

Death can also occur from status epilepticus (Question #16).

16. What is status epilepticus?

Status epilepticus is a life-threatening condition in which seizures do not stop after 30 minutes or occur one after the other without the patient recovering in between. Status epilepticus may occur in people who have never had a seizure before or in people with a known seizure disorder. There are many possible causes for status epilepticus, including brain trauma, encephalitis, meningitis, metabolic problems, toxins, and other brain problems. In people who already have epilepsy, many cases of status epilepticus are due to low blood levels of antiepileptic drugs. These episodes of status epilepticus can be prevented by making sure antiepileptic medications are taken regularly and in the proper dosage.

Prolonged seizures can injure the brain as well as cause heart, lung, and kidney problems. Patients must go to the emergency room immediately when they have status epilepticus for treatment with intravenous medication such as diazepam (Valium®), lorazepam (Ativan®), phenytoin (Dilantin®), or phenobarbital to stop the seizures. They may also require treatment for the underlying cause of the status epilepticus. If you witness a seizure that lasts longer than a couple of minutes or think the person is having status epilepticus, you should call 911.

2

WHY SO MANY TESTS?

The morning after her senior prom, Pamela fell in the bathroom as a result of her first grand mal seizure. Her mother called 911, and the ambulance took her to the nearest emergency room. By the time the doctor examined her, she was awake, but very tired and complaining of a pounding headache. Her muscles were sore, and she had bitten her tongue. Embarrassed to find herself in public dressed only in her nightgown, she wanted to go home. The doctor said she would have to stay in the hospital to have an electroencephalogram (EEG) and a magnetic resonance imaging (MRI) scan.

17. What is an EEG?

An EEG machine, or electroencephalograph, records electrical activity from your brain. Electrodes are glued or pasted to specific areas of your scalp and the machine is turned on. Amplifiers magnify the brain's tiny electrical signals. These are usually written on a large scroll of paper by sensitive pens or digitized and viewed on a computer monitor. A distinctive electrical pattern called "spike and wave" often occurs in patients with epilepsy. Other abnormalities, such as "slow waves," may indicate areas of the brain that fail to function optimally.

18. What is the purpose of an EEG?

Pamela needs an EEG (electroencephalograph) because this is her first seizure. If her EEG is normal, her doctor may choose not to give her any antiepileptic medication, hoping that the seizure was caused by a late night out (sleep deprivation). On the other hand, if there is a lot of epileptic activity, her risk of a second seizure is high.

Additionally, the pattern of spike and wave will define the seizure type. (Is the epileptic activity limited to one region of the brain, or is it widespread? Is there more than one seizure focus? What is the frequency of the spike and wave?) Determining the seizure type will help her doctor prescribe the antiepileptic medication most likely to be effective.

19. Why do I have to stay up all night before my EEG?

Sometimes your doctor will order a "sleep-deprived EEG." Fatigue tends to bring out the worst in brain waves. Many patients with epilepsy learn that sleep deprivation increases their chances of having a seizure. That is why under normal circumstances adequate rest is so important. By having you stay up all night, your doctor is maximizing the chance that epileptic activity will appear on the EEG tracing. This information will guide his choice of antiepileptic medication and help predict the likelihood of a seizure recurrence.

20. Why do they flash a bright light in my eyes during an EEG?

Photosensitive seizures occur in 2 to 14% of people with epilepsy and are more common in children. In these patients, flashing lights or changing patterns can trigger a seizure. Seizures may occur from computer games, strobe lights, television screens, or other provocative sources. One of my photosensitive patients had her first convulsion while riding in a car and looking out the window at a forest. The sunlight flashing between the trees triggered a grand mal convulsion. Luckily, she was in the back seat! In people with photosensitive epilepsy, the flashing light during the electroencephalograph (EEG), called photic stimulation, may cause a spike and wave pattern to appear on the EEG tracing or even cause a seizure. This clinches the diagnosis.

Most people with epilepsy do *not* have photosensitive seizures and can safely watch TV and play video games.

People with epilepsy who have seizures triggered by flashing lights may consider the following precautions:

1. Watch television in a well-lit room.

2. Stay at least 8 feet away from the television and use a remote control to change the channels.

3. Avoid discotheques or places with flashing lights.

4. Wear polarized sunglasses on sunny days to reduce flickering reflections.

5. Get enough sleep.

Similarly, children with photosensitive epilepsy should avoid video games, or consider the following precautions:

1. Stay as far away as practical from the video screen.

2. Don't play for more than 1 hour.

3. Play under supervision in case a seizure occurs.

21. Why do I have to hyperventilate during the EEG?

During an electroencephalograph (EEG), you may be asked to deep breathe for three to five minutes. For reasons that are not completely understood, hyperventilation lowers the seizure threshold and can bring out epileptic activity. In some patients, the EEG changes dramatically during hyperventilation, revealing more about the inner workings of the brain.

22. I already had one EEG. Why do I have to get another?

An electroencephalograph (EEG) records twenty minutes of brain activity. During a seizure, brain waves are nearly always abnormal. However, brain waves may be normal between seizures. Your doctor may order several EEGs in order to get a good look at the brain waves. I had one patient who had five normal EEGs before we finally found epileptic activity in her right temporal lobe.

23. Is there any danger when I'm hooked up to the EEG machine?

An electroencephalograph (EEG) records the brain's own electricity and consequently is very safe.

24. If I've had an EEG, why do I have to have an MRI?

An electroencephalograph (EEG) is the best way to find out about brain waves, but it does not tell much about the structural anatomy of the brain. For example, slow waves in the left temporal lobe on EEG may be the result of an old head injury. On the other hand, a brain tumor could cause the same type of EEG slowing. Clearly, the treatment for these two problems is different. Whereas no treatment might be needed for the head injury, a brain tumor might require an operation or radiation therapy.

In order to determine the cause of the abnormal EEG, your doctor needs an accurate picture of your brain. Magnetic resonance imaging (MRI) and computerized axial tomography (CAT or CT) scans are two excellent ways to see inside your brain.

25. What is the difference between an MRI and a CAT scan?

The computed axial tomography (CAT or CT) scan was the first x-ray machine to rely heavily on the computer, taking thousands of images and reconstructing them into a picture of the brain. Magnetic resonance imaging (MRI) also uses a computer, but employs a strong magnetic field instead of x-rays. CAT scans are quicker, and often better, for head injuries. MRI scans show more detail. As computers have become more sophisticated, the quality of CAT and MRI scans has improved as well.

Epilepsy specialists use the MRI to look for subtle abnormalities in the brain that can cause seizures. One of my patients with terrible memory problems had a normal CAT scan, but the MRI revealed scarring of his left temporal lobe. This abnormality was probably the cause of his seizures and memory difficulty.

Because of the MRI's strong magnet, people with cardiac pacemakers, metal heart valves, or other metal in their bodies should generally not have an MRI scan. Apart from the danger posed by metal objects, MRI technology is very safe.

26. I've been seizure-free for four years and want to stop my medication. Why does my doctor want to do another EEG?

It is extremely difficult to predict seizure recurrence. The fact that you have done well for four years is encouraging. You are probably driving and working. Your doctor is concerned you may have a seizure when you go off antiepileptic medications. Your medical history, seizure type, findings on neurological exam, brain imaging, and electroencephalograph (EEG) all go into the equation to estimate the risk of seizure recurrence.

Most neurologists believe that it is wise to continue antiepileptic medication if signs of epilepsy persist on the EEG.

This has been my experience as well. By repeating your EEG, your doctor is trying to help you make an informed decision. If your EEG is completely normal, he will probably agree to let you slowly decrease the medication dose with the goal of eventually discontinuing your antiepileptic medication. As a precaution against a possible seizure, for the first few weeks after stopping your medication, you may wish to limit driving and avoid potentially dangerous activities such as riding a bicycle, swimming, or working on a ladder or with power tools.

3

AT THE DOCTOR'S OFFICE

Everything was fine when Sally went to bed Sunday night. The next day at her office, she collapsed. Her coworkers said she let out a strange sound, fell off her chair, and her whole body jerked. She woke up in the emergency room (ER) with a throbbing headache and a sore tongue. A nurse drew her blood. Then she had an electrocardiogram (EKG) and a computed axial tomography (CAT or CT) scan. The doctor said all the tests were normal and sent her home.

On Tuesday morning, Sally was supposed to represent her department at an important meeting. Instead, she was sitting in my waiting room. While waiting to see me, Sally tried to review her presentation but couldn't concentrate.

What was the neurologist going to do, she wondered? What was wrong with her? It was a question of epilepsy, that's what the emergency room doctor said. Whatever it was, she didn't want it to happen again. How could she help the neurologist figure it out?

27. What should I expect when I go to the neurologist for the first time?

Before your visit with the neurologist, you will usually be asked to complete a screening questionnaire. You will need to list your allergies, habits (like smoking and alcohol), medications, medical problems, operations, and any illnesses in your family. Most people need to consult with other family members to get all of this information correct. It is best to review your medical history with your parents or spouse before you go to the doctor. Use the guide in Appendix A to prepare this information.

In order to understand your medical history, the doctor will ask you many important questions, either on the questionnaire or during the consultation. Here are some examples of questions you may want to ask other members of your family before you go to the doctor:

○ Were there any problems when I was born?

○ How old was I when I learned to walk and talk?

○ Was it my aunt or uncle who had seizures?

○ Did I ever have a head injury as a child?

○ Wasn't there some medication they gave me in the hospital when I had a broken leg that made me sick to my stomach?

When you provide the answers to questions like these, it will help your doctor arrive at an accurate diagnosis and appropriate treatment plan.

Additionally, there will be administrative paperwork to complete before you see the doctor. You will need to provide the name of your insurance plan if you have one. The easiest way to do this is to bring your insurance card. You will also be asked to write down your name, address, phone number, family doctor's name, and other basic information. Include a phone number of a family member or someone close to you whom you would want called if you become seriously ill.

28. What will the doctor do?

Your neurologist will begin with what doctors call a "history and physical." First, he will ask questions about your medical past to try to determine if there is an underlying cause for your seizures. For example, did you ever have a head injury, encephalitis, meningitis, or a family history of epilepsy? He will ask about your general state of health and medications to see whether these factors may have provoked a seizure. He will ask personal questions, such as whether you abuse alcohol or drugs. He will ask you to describe what you felt when you had the seizure. Some patients experience a warning, or "aura," which often is quite an unusual feeling.

When your doctor is satisfied that he has learned everything he can from talking with you, he will perform a thorough neurological examination. He will look into your eyes with a bright light, tap your reflexes, ask you to walk, maybe even hop. He will ask you to touch your finger to your nose and smile. Some of these things may seem odd. The neurological examination is the most lengthy and complex of all medical examinations. Its purpose is to complete a functional inventory of your entire central and peripheral nervous systems. It took me more than a year to learn to do it when I was a neurology resident, and I am still finding ways to do it better.

At the end of the visit, the neurologist will explain his findings. He may defer making a diagnosis until he has the results of more tests, such as an electroencephalogram (EEG) or magnetic resonance imaging (MRI) scan. He may write a prescription for antiepileptic medication and explain to you the dosage and likely side effects. In most cases, you will need to return to the office within a few weeks for a follow-up visit.

29. How long will the visit take?

For your first meeting with a neurologist, expect to spend approximately one hour with the doctor. Plan to arrive at least thirty minutes ahead of time to complete the paperwork (and find a place to park).

30. Is there anything I should bring?

All your old medical records. In Sally's case, one hopes that the emergency room doctor faxed the records to the neurologist's office. If she had a chance, it would have been worthwhile for her to go to the hospital and get her computed axial tomography (CAT or CT) scan and a copy of her emergency room sheet to bring with her.

If you have had epilepsy for a long time and have been treated by other physicians, try to make sure those records get to your new neurologist before you do. That way, your doctor will have an opportunity to review them before your visit. If you have had x-rays or electroencephalographs (EEGs), he will need these results as well. You can help a great deal in the process. I would suggest the following five steps:

1. Write a letter to your previous doctor requesting that all records, x-rays, and EEG reports be mailed to your new neurologist. Provide the address. Your letter will serve as a written release. A phone call is not sufficient. Because your medical records are confidential, they cannot be forwarded without your written consent.

2. Do not be embarrassed that you are changing doctors. New patients come to me all the time from other doctors. Sometimes patients switch because they are new in town. Sometimes they must seek a new doctor because their insurance plan has changed. In other instances, patients are not satisfied with their current doctor. Sometimes a fresh look at a case by a new doctor can result in a beneficial change in the treatment plan. (If you are not getting along with your doctor, you will probably both benefit from a change.)

3. Stop by the hospital or imaging center where your x-rays were done and get a copy of the films. Mail them to your new doctor or bring them to his office before your first appointment.

4. Call your new doctor's office a week before your appointment and check to see whether the old records arrived. If they have not, call your previous doctor and make sure they have been sent. Pick them up in person if you can.

5. Send a written request to any hospital where you have been admitted for your seizures so that these records are forwarded as well.

All these steps may sound like a lot of work, but they are often necessary to make sure the records get where they need to go. The technology of medical record keeping has lagged behind the dramatic advances in other areas of medicine. Many medical records are still transferred the old-fashioned way, by mail, on foot, or by overworked fax machines. Some doctors and hospitals have switched to electronic medical records, which allow patient information to be stored and transmitted by computer. Electronic medical records have the potential to eliminate "lost records" and reduce the legwork required to make sure your new doctor is up-to-date on all of your medical information.

In order to render a useful opinion in a complicated case, I will often spend more than an hour reviewing a patient's medical records. Then I take the x-rays to the hospital and examine them with the neuroradiologist, which takes another thirty minutes. If the case is unusual, I may need to look something up in a text-book, medical journal, or online resource, requiring another hour or so. (Don't do what some patients do. They either arrive without records ever being sent or on the day of their appointment they carry in with them piles of x-rays and pounds of photocopied pages from several different doctors, drop them on my desk, and ask, "Well, doctor, what do you think?") Although I might like to, my schedule won't permit me to spend hours reviewing records and researching a case during a patient visit.

On the other hand, when I do receive all the old records before a patient comes to see me, that first visit becomes much more exciting. I am looking forward to seeing the patient to fill in the gaps in the story. I know what has been done and how well it has been done. I know what stones still need to be turned. If I need to review the medical literature, I can do it ahead of time and be fully prepared for that new patient. My history and physical examination can be very focused and a plan of action rapidly constructed. I can spend more time explaining my diagnosis and listening to the patient's concerns. These patients get off to a running start.

31. What if my doctor asks me questions I can't (or don't want to) answer?

It always pays to be completely frank with your doctor. If you do not know whether you had febrile seizures as a child, say so. Few patients know the answers to every question. Just do your best.

Do not withhold information. For example, if the doctor asks if you drink alcohol, don't say "no" if the answer is "yes." Alcohol abuse is often associated with seizures, and it may be the cause of your problem. Misleading the doctor will result in unnecessary tests and possibly inappropriate medication, and will not help you get rid of the seizures.

An interesting story: I had two patients in the hospital with positive drug screens for marijuana. They both claimed they do not smoke the drug, but their friends do. They wanted me to believe the marijuana got into their system by passive smoking. Possible? Yes. Likely? No. Bite the bullet and tell the truth. Everything you say is confidential. Remember, your doctor is there to help you.

32. Can I bring anyone with me?

Absolutely! Please bring someone with you, not only to the doctor's office, but into the examining room. This can be a family member or close friend. Although you may be embarrassed to have someone else bear witness to your illness, that person can help you a great deal. If you can, bring someone who has seen your seizures.

Research into the doctor-patient relationship confirms that few patients remember everything that their doctor says. Many do not recall even half of what they are told. This difficulty in communication is a problem for doctors and patients in every medical field. In neurology, it may be worse, because the diseases are less common and more complicated. Doctors sometimes use language that patients cannot understand, and patients are often so anxious they do not remember what was said.

To further complicate the situation, people with epilepsy often have memory impairment, which makes it even more difficult for them to remember instructions accurately. Your companion is likely to be much calmer and more relaxed than you. You will have two sets of ears instead of one, and another mouth to ask questions.

33. How can I remember all my questions?

It pays to bring a list. Consider bringing a notebook with you to all your office visits to record your questions and your doctor's answers. (You can also write this information in Appendix A in this book.) Try to prioritize; give your doctor an opportunity to answer the most important questions. If you have a question about an article you read in a newspaper or magazine, bring it with you for your doctor to look at. I remember one patient who told me about a promising new treatment he had read about, but could not remember its name. We wasted a fair amount of time trying to figure out what it was. My patient was quite disappointed in me; certain he was missing out on a medical breakthrough. When he finally brought in the article, it was a medication I was already aware of, and it was not appropriate for him. We could have spent that time much more productively discussing the results of his electroencephalogram (EEG) and exploring the possibility of epilepsy surgery.

34. How can I remember all the answers?

Whenever I make any changes in antiepileptic medication, I give my patients my business card with written instructions on the back. If they have any questions, they can call me. When your doctor writes a new prescription, the dosage will be typed on the bottle. A few of my patients have brought tape recorders to the office to record our conversation. I discourage this practice, as it is rarely necessary.

If you are not sure what your doctor said, ask him to repeat it or write it down. Following instructions is important. In a survey of more than 800 physicians, 92 percent of them felt that compliance was an issue with their epilepsy patients. If there are reasons why you cannot follow the therapeutic plan, discuss them with your doctor. For example, there are patients who do not take their antiepileptic medication because they can't afford to get their prescription filled. No one benefits from a therapeutic plan that can't be carried out. Discuss any concerns you have regarding your diagnosis and treatment with your doctor.

35. Why doesn't my doctor spend more time with me?

Although the time with your doctor may be brief, one of the advantages of an office visit is that the physician's total focus will be on you. An office visit is an intimate experience—just you, a family member or close friend, and your doctor. In my office, there are no telephones in the examining room, and interruptions are limited to emergencies. Although there are many tasks competing for the doctor's time in a busy office, the time you spend in the examining room is completely devoted to your care. A great deal can be accomplished during this quality time.

Depending on complexity, a follow up visit takes between five and thirty minutes. This is "face-to-face" time with the physician. It does not include the hours your doctor may have spent reviewing your records and x-rays or obtaining history or other information from a referring physician or family members.

If you think you need more time with your doctor, say so. If your case is complex and there are things you do not understand, tell your doctor that you would like a longer visit. I sometimes schedule a family conference when a patient's case is difficult or they are not doing well. This provides adequate time for everyone to ask questions and thoroughly understand the problems and the treatment options.

36. Why is my doctor always late?

I schedule new patients for an hour and follow-up patients for fifteen minutes. Sometimes I finish a new patient in forty-five minutes, sometimes it takes an hour and a half. A follow-up can be as brief as five minutes or as long as thirty minutes. The plan is for it all to equal out by the end of the day. Sometimes it works, but frequently the plan fails. When I run late, I don't like it, but it happens. I don't want to rush through anyone's visit, and if new problems come up, they need to be addressed. I would much prefer to finish on time.

I remember one patient who was angry with me because I was an hour late for his appointment. Unfortunately, he didn't tell me. He was sullen during the visit and didn't tell me much about his problems with his seizures. At the end of the visit, he suddenly began to rant and rave about how inconsiderate I was to waste his valuable time. It was late in the afternoon on a busy day, and I didn't even know I was behind schedule. I wish he had told me sooner so I could have apologized and gotten on with the visit. As it was, we didn't accomplish much and neither one of us was very happy. (Listening to him complain took even more time, and my next patient wasn't happy either.)

The busier your doctor is, the more likely he will be off schedule. It is best to prepare for this. Assume he will be late. Bring a book or office paperwork with you to your appointment. If you can, leave children at home with a babysitter or friend. Trying to control energetic kids in a busy waiting room can be fatiguing.

If your doctor tends to run late, there is something you can do. Explain to the scheduling secretary that this is a problem for you and ask for the earliest appointment in the morning or the first one after lunch. Your doctor is more likely to be prompt for these appointments. If that doesn't help, you might check around for another doctor!

37. What do I need to bring to a follow-up visit?

In order to help you manage your seizures, there is a mini-mum of information your doctor needs at every visit. He needs to know your history and findings of your physical and neurological examination, as well as results of any testing you may have had, such as magnetic resonance imaging (MRI) or electroencephalo-graphs (EEGs). All of this information has already been collected during your initial consultation and will be in your chart.

You need to provide two additional pieces of information at each visit. First is the number of seizures you have had. I recom-mend a seizure calendar. I give each patient a seizure calendar that is good for six months, but you can use any kind of calendar you want. (There is one in Appendix A.) I have very few patients who can recall how many seizures they have had without writing them down. And remember, it doesn't do the doctor any good if you keep a seizure calendar and leave it stuck on the refrigerator! (I heard that one yesterday.) Bring it with you. Second, your doc-tor needs to know which antiepileptic medication you are taking and the correct dose. The easiest thing to do is to bring the bottles with you. If you are taking any other medications or alternative treatments such as vitamins or herbs, bring those bottles, too.

38. How can I get the most out of an office visit?

First of all, don't be late. The time reserved for you will disappear if you are not there. If your doctor has other appointments following yours, your visit will likely be cut short.

If you have small children, find someone to look after them while you are with the doctor. You won't be able to pay attention to a crying baby and your doctor's technical explanation about your seizures at the same time!

Because time with your doctor is limited, it is critical to know how to use it to your advantage. The worst thing you can do is wait for the visit to be nearly over, then tell the doctor that you have just started getting these terrible headaches, or pull out a list of things that have been bothering you. If you present your doctor with a new complaint, he will likely have to perform a more extensive examination than he was anticipating. A complete neurological examination can take fifteen minutes or a lot longer, depending on the problem and the patient. He may also have to review your chart, looking for similar symptoms you may have had in the past. Again, this will take time. Most medical records are not computerized, and it can take many minutes to locate information in a thick chart.

If you wait until the end of your visit to get to the real reason why you are there, you have placed your doctor in an impossible position. If he is like me, there is a waiting room full of patients, and he doesn't want to apologize to them for the rest of the day because he is running late. On the other hand, in order to treat your new problem appropriately, he will need to review your chart and perform a neurological examination. He wants to take proper care of everyone, and now he's in a bind.

When you see your neurologist, say hello, then tell him why you are there. For example, "Doctor, I haven't seen you for six months, and I'm here for a check-up." Or, "Doctor, I saw you three months ago, but that medicine doesn't really agree with my stomach, and my seizures are no better." Better yet, "Doctor, that new medication I started yesterday gave me a rash, so I came right in. Take a look at these welts!" If you can help your doctor focus on your problem, you will get the best advantage of his time and skill. He will appreciate your forthrightness and you will get a better result. Teamwork with your doctor is your goal.

39. Why do I have to bring my medication with me if the doctor has all the information in the chart?

I used to wonder this myself. Interestingly, there are many variables that determine the type of antiepileptic medication and dose a patient actually takes. Although I record this information in each patient's chart at every visit, it never ceases to amaze me how often what I have written down does not agree with what the patient tells me at the next visit. I have learned from experience that there are a number of factors that can cause this problem:

○ The patient does not understand verbal instructions. This happens from time to time. Now, when I make a change in dosage or antiepileptic medication, I write it down on my business card and hand it to the patient. This usually works.

○ Second, there was confusion over dosing. Many pills come in different strengths. Divalproex sodium (Depakote®), for example, comes in 250-mg and 500-mg sizes. There is an extended-release formulation as well. I have had quite a few patients who did not know which dose they were on. One patient knew she was taking five pills, but for months we could never determine whether she was taking 1,250 mg or 2,500 mg. Even though the pills are different colors, we still could not figure it out! (This became a problem when she needed a refill.) Finally, she brought the pills to the office and we determined her dose.

○ Sometimes the drug dosage is adjusted over the phone between visits. Although these changes are supposed to be entered into the chart, this does not always happen. One reason is that sometimes the change is made by another physician. This may happen over the phone at night when the chart is not available, or during a visit to the hospital or emergency room.

○ The patient is not taking the prescribed dosage because the prescription was not filled properly. Mistakes by pharmacists are rare. More frequently, certain pills are not available, such as the 30-mg size of phenytoin (Dilantin®), and the prescription isn't filled.

○ The patient tried the new dose, but developed symptoms of toxicity and went back to the old dose without telling the doctor. This happens all the time. If you need to make a change, inform your doctor. Don't wait until the next visit to tell him you're not doing what he thinks you're doing. Remember that communication between you and your doctor is essential to good patient care.

When you bring all your medications with you, your doctor can see which drugs have been prescribed by other physicians. Some of these may interact with the ones you are taking or with one he is thinking of prescribing. When you bring your bottles with you, it provides a double check to ensure that both you and your doctor know the name and dose of all your medications. Don't leave home without them!

40. I keep running out of medication and have to call the office for a refill. I seem to spend a lot of time "on hold." What can I do?

In order to refill a prescription over the phone, your chart has to be pulled by someone in medical records and reviewed by the doctor, and the pharmacy has to be called. If the doctor is at the hospital or with patients, he will not be able to attend to it right away. If you have recently been seen in the office, your office note is likely in the transcription department being typed and the chart may be difficult to locate.

In order to avoid running out of antiepileptic medication, the best thing to do is to check how much medication you have left before you visit the doctor. It is much easier for him to write a refill prescription while you and your chart are together. At each office visit, I try to ask patients if they need a refill, but I don't always remember. If you do need a new prescription, it is preferable to call during business hours. Some patients seem to think they cannot refill their prescription until there are absolutely no pills left in the bottle. (This is not true.) Then they call at midnight, desperate because they have run out. Try to avoid this awkward situation by planning ahead. Your doctor will appreciate it.

41. Is there anyone besides my doctor who can explain things to me?

Your doctor will try to answer questions about your disease, medications, tests, and prognosis. Some questions, such as how to obtain assistance in purchasing medication or arranging transportation, may be better answered by a social worker, nurse, or a staff member in the doctor's office. You and your family may benefit from an instructional videotape or epilepsy support group. In-depth information can be found in several excellent books (see the Bibliography) and educational pamphlets listed in the Epilepsy Foundation catalog. Another excellent educational resource is www.epilepsy.com (Appendix H).

If you think you need more information, ask your doctor to refer you to a comprehensive epilepsy center where many of these services will be available to you. There are more than 100 epilepsy centers in the United States that specialize in the treatment of patients with difficult to control seizures (Appendix D).

42. I have several doctors. How can I make sure they are all working together?

In these days of specialized medical care, many patients have two or more physicians. In fact, all of my patients have a primary care physician. Some patients even have other neurologists in their hometowns. A large number of my patients see psychiatrists, who also prescribe medication, typically for depression or anxiety, which are common problems in people with epilepsy.

When a patient's case is complex, I make sure that a copy of my dictated office note is sent to the other doctors involved. This process can be facilitated if you bring the business cards of your other doctors with you, so the name and address is clear. (I sometimes have patients request that their notes be sent to their other neurologist, but they don't know who he is!) Remember, good communication leads to good results.

4

MEDICATIONS

For the last three months, Gloria's seizures had gone out of control. She dutifully recorded each one in her seizure calendar and telephoned me every month. With each call, I increased the dose of her antiepileptic medication by one-half a tablet. Two weeks ago, she ran out of medication and refilled her prescription at a new pharmacy close to home.

Today, she sat in my office as an emergency work-in, so dizzy she could barely walk. She couldn't focus her eyes and felt sick to her stomach. I opened her chart to see which medication she was taking and asked her the dose. She couldn't remember, so I asked to see the bottle.

When Gloria pulled the plastic bottle out of her purse, she squirmed in her chair. She knew I had told her to take the brand name medication, not the generic. But the brand name was too expensive, she thought, more than fifty cents a pill, and she had to take six of them a day. She couldn't afford it, but was too embarrassed to say anything.

When I saw that the bottle contained round white pills, not the thin pink ones, I asked why she hadn't followed instructions. Despite her blurred vision, Gloria could see I was frustrated and annoyed. She began crying and stumbled out of the room. She told herself she'd have to find a better neurologist, one who was more sympathetic and could really help with her seizures. Initially, I was perplexed. Why didn't Gloria follow instructions? Didn't she know I thought the brand name drug was necessary for her difficult to control seizures?

43. Why should I take the brand name medication if the generic contains the same active ingredient and costs less?

Sometimes a generic antiepileptic drug is adequate. However, it may not be appropriate for people with difficult to control seizures. The Food and Drug Administration (FDA) allows a range of 80 to 125% in bioequivalence from the brand name preparation, so although generics are similar, they are not the same.

In addition, although the active ingredient in each pill or capsule may be identical to the brand name preparation, the amount of antiepileptic medication absorbed and the rate at which it is taken up by the body may not be identical. This variability between brands and the generic may be the reason Gloria became toxic on her medication. The last batch of pills she bought at the new pharmacy was better absorbed and gave her a higher drug level.

For some patients, these differences may not matter. Constant drug levels may be less critical for patients whose seizures respond easily to medication and do not require frequent dosage adjustments. But for patients with difficult to control epilepsy, many physicians have observed that the difference in the amount of active ingredient combined with the difference in preparation can result in breakthrough seizures. Changes in drug level may also cause toxic side effects. Many patients who are switched from the brand name to generic antiepileptic medication end up switching back.

When patients suffer persistent seizures, I recommend brand name antiepileptic medication so that we have a better chance to obtain consistent, effective blood levels. Generic medication is not cost effective when it results in breakthrough seizures or side effects requiring extra office visits, trips to the emergency room, hospitalizations, or other expensive treatments.

Had Gloria brought her husband with her, he could have explained that she bought the generic medication because of financial constraints. He would have calmed her down, and the office visit could have turned into a productive one.

If a generic drug is the only practical option, it may be more successful if you always take pills made by the same manufacturer since the differences from lot to lot by the same manufacturer may be less than the differences between different preparations from different manufacturers. When your prescription is refilled, make sure the color and shape of the pills have not changed and ask the pharmacist if they are from the same company.

The American Academy of Neurology recently (2007) published a Position Statement opposing generic substitution without the patient's and their doctor's consent.* Along these lines, the state of Tennessee passed a law requiring pharmacists to notify physicians and patients prior to an antiepileptic drug switch from one manufacturer to another. Several other states have laws limiting the substitution of generics for brand name medication. Advocacy by the Epilepsy Foundation and others to pass laws that protect patients from potentially dangerous substitution of generic drugs is ongoing. The FDA certifies generics as equally bioavailable, but many doctors and persons with epilepsy report stories like Gloria's. Until further research settles the issue of generic drug equivalence to brand, substitution of a generic for a brand antiepileptic medication should only be undertaken after careful consideration and under your physician's supervision.

44. My doctor keeps writing prescriptions for these new epilepsy drugs, but I can't afford them! What can I do?

Based on my experience, your doctor is probably preoccupied with the complex medical decision making required to treat your

---

*Liow K, Barkley GL, Pollard JR, et al. Position statement on the coverage of anticonvulsant drugs for the treatment of epilepsy. Neurology 2007;68:1249–1250.

epilepsy and maximize your overall quality of life rather than thinking about whether you can actually afford the antiepileptic medication.

Of course, both are important. One of my patients told me he was taking a dose lower than I had prescribed because of side effects. When I pressed him for details, he eventually admitted the drug was too expensive and he couldn't pay for the full dose. Several of the newer antiepileptic drugs may cost as much as four dollars a pill, and more than one pill may be required each day. The cost of one of these antiepileptic medications may add up to several hundred dollars per month.

If you cannot afford the prescribed medication, tell your doctor. There are a number of ways he may be able to help you:

○ He may have free samples that can get you started for several days. If you do not tolerate the medication, at least you will not have invested money for a whole month's supply.

○ He may be able to enroll you in a patient assistance program. Many patients with epilepsy have difficulty affording antiepileptic drugs. Because of this problem, most manufacturers of antiepileptic drugs provide medication at no charge for a limited time. Eligibility is determined by the company. A form must be completed by your physician and sent to the pharmaceutical company to enroll you in the program. (I have filled out many of these forms!) Three helpful websites that provide information on patient assistance programs are: www.rxhope.com, www.needymeds.com, and www.access2wellness.com. Contact information for pharmaceutical companies is provided in Appendix B.

○ Your doctor can refer you to a social worker who may find other types of financial support for you, such as Medicare or Medicaid. Many of my patients receive financial assistance.

○ Your doctor can change the prescription to a low-cost drug such as phenobarbital if he thinks it will be effective. Phenobarbital is inexpensive and needs only be taken once or twice a day, but it also has numerous drug interactions and may cause adverse effects such as sleepiness and slowed thinking.

○ Join a local epilepsy support group. Remember, you are not alone. Epilepsy is a common disorder affecting almost 1% of the population. Chances are other members of the support group have already located the pharmacies in town with the best prices. The Epilepsy Foundation can help you find local resources.

45. Why does epilepsy medication cost so much?

It is hard to imagine a tiny pill being worth three or four dollars. This adds up to a lot of money if you take many of them each day. In my research in antiepileptic drug development, I have had the opportunity to work closely with pharmaceutical companies that manufacture antiepileptic drugs. Each new drug must be shown to be safe and effective before it can be approved by the Food and Drug Administration (FDA) (Chapter 14).

Most experimental drugs never succeed in reaching the marketplace, driving up the cost of the ones that do. It takes ten to fifteen years of hard work by clinical investigators (and patients!) and hundreds of millions of dollars to bring a new drug to market. The price of your antiepileptic medication reflects these high developmental costs.

46. What is the best drug for seizure control and overall quality of life?

When I prescribe a new antiepileptic medication, I have to choose the appropriate drug for the seizure type, decide whether it will be used alone (monotherapy) or in combination with other antiepileptic drugs (polytherapy), take into account possible drug interactions with other medications the patient may be taking, estimate the right dose for the patient's body size and metabolism, and devise an easily tolerated dosing schedule.

There are more than a dozen commonly used antiepileptic drugs. (See Appendix B for generic and brand names.) The best drug for seizure control is the one that stops your seizures with the lowest dose and causes the fewest side effects.

Sometimes the first drug I prescribe does the trick. However, because every patient is different, a drug that works for one patient may not work for another, or side effects may occur in one patient that did not occur in another. Consequently, finding the "best" drug is a combination of medical expertise and luck.

The new science of pharmacogenomics is helping to predict how certain individuals will respond to specific drugs. Eventually, when we fully understand a person's genetic makeup, we should be able to predict the most effective and best-tolerated antiepileptic drug for that individual's specific metabolism and type of epilepsy. Pharmacogenomics may ultimately eliminate much of the trial and error that constitutes a large part of today's clinical epilepsy care.

47. What do I do if I forget a dose of medication?

In general, my advice is to make it up. Otherwise it may take several days for your drug level to return to normal. However, if your next dose is due within an hour or two, you are likely to develop toxic symptoms such as nausea or dizziness if you take the pills so close together. In that case, it's better to resume your schedule and make up the missed dose three to four hours after your next dose.

If you frequently forget your antiepileptic medication, there are simple techniques to help you remember. Try taking your medication at specific times of day or in conjunction with certain activities (i.e., breakfast, brushing your teeth, going to bed). Alarms, pill boxes, and other devices may help (Question #13).

48. Why do I have to get antiepileptic drug levels?

Because of differences in body size and metabolism, it is difficult to predict the exact dose to prescribe for each patient. Drug levels allow the doctor to monitor how much antiepileptic medication is in your system at a given time.

When one of my patients has a seizure, I often order a drug level. If the level is low, I will increase the dose to achieve better seizure control. If, on the other hand, the level is high, I am more inclined to switch to a different antiepileptic medication.

When patients complain of symptoms such as dizziness or clumsiness, I order a drug level to see whether the medication is responsible. If the level is high, it's likely that the symptoms are due to the medication, so I lower the dose and wait for the patient to improve. If the level is low, the patient's symptoms are likely due to another neurological problem that requires further investigation.

Drug levels are also a useful way to monitor compliance. Jan complained of daily seizures despite a combination of phenytoin (Dilantin®) and divalproex sodium (Depakote®). When I checked the levels of these drugs in her blood, both were zero! It didn't take a medical degree to figure out why the medications were not working.

49. Why do I have to take medication three times a day?

The purpose of spreading doses throughout the day is to maintain a constant blood level. After you swallow a pill, your body absorbs it and proceeds to break it down and excrete it. The speed of this process varies in different people. Additionally, some antiepileptic medications last longer in the body than others. Phenobarbital, for example, is metabolized slowly and can be taken in one daily dose. Carbamazepine (Tegretol®) is metabolized more rapidly, and ideally should be taken three times a day. The more difficult seizures are to control, the more important it is to maintain a steady blood level throughout the day. Frequent doses of antiepileptic medication or switching to an extended-release preparation may improve seizure control.

50. My medication dose keeps increasing. Am I becoming immune to my medication?

A phenomenon called "autoinduction" can occur with carbamazepine (Tegretol®). In essence, the body learns to metabolize the drug more effectively. Consequently, a higher dose may be required to maintain the same drug level after several weeks of use.

51. Will I have to take this medication forever?

Many children outgrow their epilepsy and will no longer require antiepileptic medication. Some adults become seizure-free after their first or second seizure, and their medication can often be successfully discontinued. On the other hand, if you are an adult and have had seizures for many years, you will probably do worse without antiepileptic medication. When patients are seizure-free for a few years, it is reasonable to reassess the medication strategy and consider decreasing and eventually discontinuing the antiepileptic treatment depending upon the patient's preference, antiepileptic medication tolerance, results of electroencephalogram and magnetic resonance imaging, and other factors.

With continued medical progress, more effective treatments with fewer side effects will likely become available in the future. Many new antiepileptic drugs are under development (Appendix B).

5

MEDICATION SIDE EFFECTS

A week after I prescribed a new antiepileptic medication for Janet, she called the office. I had warned her that a rash was one of the potential side effects of her new medication, and now she had one. Her husband had noticed large, red blotches on her back. I asked her to come to the office so that I could see it. Upon examination that afternoon, I found three saucer-shaped areas on her back about five inches in diameter. There were none on her face, chest, or arms. This was not a typical drug reaction. I sent her to the dermatologist to be sure.

Janet was happy with the cream the dermatologist gave her. After a week of applying it four times a day, the rash went away. It seems she had a fungal infection on her back, something like athlete's foot. Because this wasn't a drug reaction, I didn't have to change her antiepileptic medication, and her seizures have been controlled.

52. What else can cause a rash besides a new drug?

In Janet's case, it was a fungal infection. I remember one patient who complained of a rash on his legs after he began a new antiepileptic medication; he turned out to have flea bites. Another patient complained of a rash on her face, which was adolescent acne. I used to assume that all rashes were related to medications, but now I insist on seeing the patient before I make changes in therapy.

53. What should I do if I break out in a rash?

Approximately one out of every six patients will develop a rash due to an antiepileptic drug. The risk of a rash from an antiepileptic drug varies depending upon the type of drug and your medical history. For example, rashes are more common with carbamazepine (Tegretol®), lamotrigine (Lamictal®), and phenytoin (Dilantin®), but less common with divalproex sodium (Depakote®), gabapentin (Neurontin®), and levetiracetam (Keppra®). In addition, you are more likely to develop a rash if you have had one in the past, even if it was from a different anti-epileptic drug. If you develop a rash from an antiepileptic drug, this is a type of drug allergy. Make sure you tell your doctor if you have drug allergies to any other kind of medication.

If you develop a rash, call your doctor immediately. In many cases, you will be asked to stop the medication. Allergic reactions often start with a rash, but may evolve into more serious medical problems. In certain circumstances, your doctor may wish to continue the medication. I usually ask my patients to come to the office so that I can see the rash, assess its severity, determine whether it is due to an antiepileptic drug, and decide upon the best course of action for that particular patient. If I'm not sure, I'll send the patient to a dermatologist for a more informed diagnosis. Most antiepileptic drug rashes occur within a few weeks after you start taking the medication, are mild, and do not lead to severe complications.

54. What is a "potential" side effect?

If you read about your antiepileptic medication on the internet, in the *Physicians' Desk Reference* (PDR), or on the fact sheet provided by your pharmacist, you will be confronted with a long list of frightening side effects. These are problems that the drug has the *potential* to cause. It is your doctor's responsibility to be aware of these, which is why they are listed in the PDR, a thick reference book written for physicians. You may develop one or more of these complications or may not develop any of them. They are *possible* side effects, not probable ones.

55. After I get out of bed and take my first dose of medication, I always get dizzy and see double. By late morning, the symptoms go away. What can I do?

Dizziness and double vision are common symptoms of antiepileptic drug toxicity. You have identified exactly when they occur, which will help your doctor fix the problem. (This is a good example illustrating how a seizure calendar, which includes not only your seizures, but your side effects, menstrual period, times you missed medication, and other important information, can help you and your doctor manage your epilepsy.)

To get rid of your dizziness, the obvious first choice is to lower the morning dosage of your antiepileptic medication. However, this may not be possible if you need the large dose to control your seizures. In that case, try spreading out the pills. For example, instead of two pills when you wake up, take one, followed by the second pill at 10:00 AM. In this manner, you will take the same daily amount, but will avoid toxic side effects caused by a high blood level. Another approach is to take the two pills with breakfast, which may slow the medication's absorption and prevent the "peak" side effects.

You may also wish to consider an extended-release product, such as Carbatrol®, Tegretol XR®, or Depakote ER®. Extended-release products eliminate the high peaks that may occur soon after taking your antiepileptic medication and also prevent the "trough" levels from dipping too low.

56. I've gained so much weight since I started my new medication! Why did that happen?

Up to half the patients taking divalproex sodium (Depakote®) gain weight, sometimes large amounts. The drug causes increased appetite, which results in increased weight. Other metabolic mechanisms may also be involved. A combination of a healthy diet with the appropriate amount of calories and regular exercise may correct the problem. If the weight gain is severe, you may need to switch to another antiepileptic drug.

Carbamazepine (Tegretol®), gabapentin (Neurontin®), and pregabalin (Lyrica®) may also cause weight gain. Certain other antiepileptic drugs, such as felbamate (Felbatol®), topiramate (Topamax®), and zonisamide (Zonegran®) tend to cause weight loss. These effects vary quite a bit between patients. Discuss your concerns regarding weight gain or loss with your doctor. Together, you can choose an antiepileptic drug that will influence your weight in the desired direction.

57. My doctor wanted to switch me from one antiepileptic medication to another. But after the first dose I was too dizzy to stand up. What happened?

Replacing one drug with another may be difficult. Frequently, undesirable interactions occur between drugs. For example, when phenytoin (Dilantin®) is added to divalproex sodium (Depakote®), the effective phenytoin level can become too high. The same dose of phenytoin without divalproex sodium would not cause symptoms. When a new antiepileptic drug is added to your regimen, it is often advisable to decrease the dose of the previous medication. Although lowering the dose of one drug risks a seizure, it can prevent toxicity from drug interactions.

Switching drugs is a delicate balancing act. During this process, stay in close contact with your doctor and report any symptoms of toxicity or breakthrough seizures.

58. Do I have to live with all these side effects? They're worse than the epilepsy!

They shouldn't be. There is now a large assortment of effective antiepileptic drugs for you and your doctor to try (Appendix B). These medications work by employing one or more different pharmacological mechanisms and have different side effect profiles. For example, as discussed in Question #56, some drugs may cause weight gain, while others may cause weight loss. Certain antiepileptic drugs are also beneficial for other medical problems, such as headache or mood disorders. If you suffer from one of these conditions, it might be wise to choose an antiepileptic drug that may help both your epilepsy and the other disorder. Discuss your concerns about side effects and other health issues with your doctor and try and choose the antiepileptic drug that is best for you.

59. Someone told me phenobarbital is addicting. Is that true?

Phenobarbital, primidone (Mysoline®), and mephobarbital (Mebaral®) are barbiturates that may be habit forming. However, they can be excellent, low-cost medications to control seizures. I have used these drugs with very good results in my practice.

Because the body develops physiological tolerance to these medications, unpleasant withdrawal symptoms can occur if you suddenly stop taking one of these antiepileptic drugs. You may experience a fast heart rate, tremor, or even withdrawal seizures. In order to prevent these symptoms, always taper these medications slowly before discontinuing them. Do not run out.

Last week, one of my patients stopped her primidone (Mysoline®) abruptly and developed status epilepticus (Question #16). It corrected as soon as we gave her some phenobarbital in the emergency room.

60. Can antiepileptic medications affect my sex life?

Some antiepileptic drugs can cause impotence in men. Decreased libido and impotence are significantly more frequent with phenobarbital and primidone (Mysoline®) than with other antiepileptic drugs. Antiepileptic drugs may also adversely affect the sex life of women.

Although these problems are of a personal nature, your physician cannot help unless you discuss them. Recently, awareness of women's health issues has increased dramatically, both among patients and their physicians. Don't be shy about mentioning your problems. You may find it easier to bring up these issues with the doctor's nurse before you see the doctor. In addition, women should alert their gynecologists if they are taking antiepileptic medications. This is very important if you are using the birth control pill or other hormonal contraception (Questions #131 and #132).

61. My doctor told me he had to do blood tests every year to check for side effects. What are they?

Some patients develop abnormalities due to certain antiepileptic drugs. For example, carbamazepine (Tegretol®) can lower the number of white blood cells, and divalproex sodium (Depakote®) can lower the number of blood platelets. Rarely the white blood cell count becomes too low to fight infection and the carbamazepine must be discontinued. Similarly, if the platelet count drops too low, the blood will not clot properly, and bleeding may occur. Consequently, the divalproex sodium may have to be discontinued.

Many antiepileptic drugs may cause abnormalities in liver function. These are usually not severe. However, if they are, the dose must be decreased or the medication discontinued.

By periodically monitoring your white blood cell count, platelet count, and liver function and performing other tests, your doctor can keep an eye on possible medication side effects. The type of blood tests ordered and how often they are performed depends upon which antiepileptic drug you are taking, your own medical history, and your physician's judgment. Your doctor's goal is to detect any abnormalities and make the necessary changes in your antiepileptic medication before symptoms occur.

6

ALTERNATIVE THERAPY

Danny's mother was an actress. Her seizure disorder was well controlled with phenytoin (Dilantin®). She didn't like taking the medication, because she had grown accustomed to herbal therapies. However, since she had been seizure-free for many years, she was reluctant to stop taking the antiepileptic medication. Seizures were not a new phenomenon in her life, as her uncle also had seizures. She was conflicted by her belief in herbal alternative therapies and her obvious benefits from taking the phenytoin.

Danny was only a "C" student in school, but was artistically talented like his mother. He attended a special school for the arts. Danny had a febrile convulsion at age three, but developed normally without further seizures. However, a month after his sixteenth birthday, he had five brief generalized tonic clonic seizures in a three-week period.

Due to the irregular nature of her work, Danny's mother didn't have health insurance and didn't take him to a physician. Because she was a firm believer in alternative therapies, she gave him herbal medications, some from her own organic garden. For a few months, the homegrown treatments seemed to work. Then Danny had another convulsion, this time at the mall, resulting in an ambulance ride to the emergency room. The following day, she brought Danny to see me.

Danny's neurological examination was normal, but his electroencephalogram (EEG) revealed generalized spike and wave at three to four cycles per second, suggesting a genetically inherited epilepsy. It took me a while to convince Danny and his mother that a conventional antiepileptic drug such as divalproex sodium (Depakote®), in spite of its potential side effects, would help Danny more than backyard herbs. Two years after beginning the divalproex sodium, Danny remains seizure-free.

62. What were some nonscientific treatments for epilepsy?

Hippocrates (460 to 337 BC) wrote the first scientific paper on epilepsy, *On the Sacred Disease.* He recognized that epilepsy was a disease of the brain due to physical causes. Hippocrates recommended that epilepsy be treated, "not by magic, but by diet and drugs."

Nonetheless, an impressive number of useless and unpleasant therapies have been inflicted on people with epilepsy since then. Here are a few examples: eat a raven's egg or a frog's liver, eat a pigeon and drink its blood, eat a wing-ant, drink a gladiator's blood and eat his liver, and kill a dog and drink its bile. Innocent bystanders could be helpful, too—the person who first saw the patient have a convulsion should urinate into his shoe, stir it, and give it to the patient to drink!

In 1954, Herbert Jasper wrote that the scientific advances made by Hughlings Jackson, William Gowers, and others would lead to "hope" and "more rational therapy" for the person with epilepsy. Modern science has enabled us to move beyond ancient and unproven remedies. (If you have to have epilepsy, it is definitely better to have it now than at any time in the past.)

63. Are there any natural treatments for epilepsy?

The first effective anticonvulsant drug, bromide, is a derivative of the naturally occurring element bromine. Bromide is not often used today because of its side effects and the ready availability of less toxic antiepileptic drugs. No other natural treatment has been proven effective for the treatment of epilepsy.

64. Aren't natural treatments healthier?

The fact that a substance is "natural" does not guarantee either its effectiveness or its safety. Arsenic is a naturally occurring metallic element that can cause anemia, cramps, diarrhea, malignant skin tumors, and paralysis. It was used as a poison gas in World War I. These facts, however, did not keep arsenic from being included as one of the main ingredients in a now forgotten antiepileptic concoction prescribed in the 1930s.

65. Can I control seizures with vitamins?

One type of epilepsy is caused by a deficiency of pyridoxine (vitamin B6). This seizure disorder is rare and usually diagnosed in infancy. Unfortunately, pyridoxine is not useful in treating other forms of epilepsy.

Taking megavitamins has not been shown to help control seizures. Too much of certain vitamins can be harmful.

Very low levels of magnesium and calcium can trigger seizures, but these conditions are infrequent. Patients without a deficiency of these two minerals are unlikely to achieve better seizure control by taking either a calcium or magnesium supplement.

66. What about herbal medications?

No herbs, oils, or potions have been proven to help control seizures. On the other hand, some herbal medicines may have a scientific basis for seizure control.

Herbal medicine has been used in China for more than two thousand years. The Chinese herb tian ma is commonly used for the treatment of epilepsy. Qingyangshen is another traditional Chinese medicine that may have antiepileptic properties. Laboratory experiments have shown that a combination of phenytoin and qingyangshen affects gene expression in the brain and reduce seizures in epileptic rats.

A Japanese epilepsy drug, shosaiko-to-go-keishi-ka-shakuyaku-to, an extract of nine herbs, consists of many known and unknown substances. This preparation has been reported to control seizures in patients. In the laboratory, it can inhibit convulsions in a type of epilepsy-prone mouse.

It is likely that additional useful prescription drugs will be developed from plants and animals. Nature's gardens have already produced drugs for congestive heart failure, high blood pressure, leukemia, muscle cramps, and pain control. Pharmaceutical companies are not blind to the value of naturally occurring medicines. Approximately 25% of all prescriptions contain at least one active ingredient from plants.

As yet undiscovered plant species exist in the oceans and rain forests that may also prove to have therapeutic potential. New research efforts are currently directed toward these promising alternative therapies.

The Food and Drug Administration (FDA) has recognized that useful medications may be obtained from plants and approved the first botanical prescription drug in October 2006 (for warts!). More than 300 other botanicals are pending review. Many more botanicals, perhaps some for epilepsy, are sure to be developed in the near future.

67. Why not use herbal medication? Can it do any harm?

There are five significant problems with herbal and other alternative therapies:

1. Despite promotional claims, these drugs have generally not received approval by the Food and Drug Administration (FDA). When an antiepileptic medication has been approved by the FDA, you can be confident that it has been extensively tested in animals and human beings at a cost of many millions of dollars. The manufacturer must produce a product with known and consistent ingredients, a profile of expected

side effects, specific indications for use, and expected benefits. Herbal remedies available at the health food store are not subjected to this rigorous testing or these strict manufacturing standards. They may be helpful, useless, or dangerous.

2. Herbal medications may have harmful side effects. An example is the Chinese herb ma huang (herbal ecstasy), which is purported to produce a feeling that all is right and good with the world. Evaluation of this natural therapy by the FDA suggests caution because this drug can cause heart attacks and seizures.

   Other herbal medications that may be dangerous include ginkgo biloba, which may cause seizures, and kava kava, which may cause liver failure.

3. Another limitation of traditional medications is that the ingredients are not labeled. You may be allergic to the contents and not know it.

4. Herbal medicines may interact with prescription drugs, resulting in unwanted side effects. For example, St. John's wort, commonly used for depression, may increase the metabolism of the birth control pill, rendering it ineffective and resulting in unwanted pregnancies. It may also interact with cyclosporine, an immunosuppressive drug used in transplant patients, resulting in organ rejection. Because of the possibility of drug-drug interactions, if you are taking alternative therapies (and many people with epilepsy do), make sure you share this information with your doctor. If your doctor knows what you are taking, then you both can evaluate the risks and benefits of your alternative medicine and come up with a rational treatment plan.

5. Perhaps the most persuasive argument against alternative medications is that they can prevent someone from taking a known, effective medication. Based on Danny's strong family history of epilepsy, his normal neurological examination, and

the epileptic pattern on his electroencephalogram, I diagnosed a genetic epilepsy likely to respond to divalproex sodium (Depakote®) or other antiepileptic drugs such as lamotrigine (Lamictal®) or topiramate (Topamax®). His mother's belief in herbal medicine resulted in his having more seizures than necessary, certainly not what she desired for her child. Had Danny come to see me sooner, we could have controlled his seizures and spared him a frightening and expensive trip to the emergency room.

At the very least, rather than alternative therapy, these unproven approaches to treatment should be considered complementary or additional to proven therapies.

68. What about biofeedback?

Biofeedback is a group of techniques in which people attempt to consciously control involuntary body functions, such as heart rate, blood pressure, or their brain waves. A heart monitor or brain wave machine, for example, provides instant biofeedback of the results. There are reports of seizure control with biofeedback. In one study, patients practiced meditation for twenty minutes each day for a year. They experienced significant brain wave changes as well as a decrease in the duration and frequency of their seizures. Biofeedback is rarely used in the treatment of epilepsy and has not been well studied. It appears to help some people and has no known side effects. A trial of biofeedback should be considered by highly motivated patients.

69. What about acupuncture?

Acupuncture has been used in both canine and human epilepsy. Acupressure has also been tried to control seizures. There is one report from Anhui Province in China of prompt control of status epilepticus with acupuncture. The Food and Drug Administration (FDA) has reclassified acupuncture needles from Class III to Class II devices. This new category removes the "investigational use" labeling requirement and may facilitate increased use of this procedure. It is hoped that more research on the effectiveness of acupuncture for epilepsy will be performed as well.

70. Can't I control epilepsy with diet?

Two diets, the ketogenic and modified Atkins, may be successful in controlling seizures (Chapter 11).

71. Can any lifestyle changes help control seizures?

John had a brain tumor removed from his left temporal lobe five years ago. He had no seizures for the first six months after surgery, but then they returned. About once every two weeks, he would have a convulsion. Despite trials of several new antiepileptic medications, he continued to have breakthrough seizures.

I admitted John to the hospital to take a closer look at his seizures on our electroencephalographic and video monitoring equipment (EEG/CCTV). Despite sleep deprivation and withdrawal of his medications, John did not have a single seizure in 17 days of inpatient monitoring. After repeated interviews about his social habits, John finally admitted to the neuropsychologist that he tended to drink a few beers every two weeks. It was at this time he had his seizures. Many patients can drink alcohol without endangering their seizure control, but others cannot. Modification of alcohol intake, including beer, may make a difference in seizure control.

Caffeine stimulates the brain and is an ingredient in coffee, tea, and many soft drinks. Most patients tolerate these beverages without difficulty, but excessive amounts of caffeine can lower the seizure threshold and result in a breakthrough seizure. If you drink more than a few cups of coffee or cans of soda a day, consider cutting back or switching to a decaffeinated brand. This may help with seizure control.

Another important lifestyle factor in seizure control is adequate rest. Whether it is teenagers staying up late to study (or party), pregnant women who cannot sleep, or busy executives with pressing deadlines, seizures can result from sleep deprivation. For many people, a good night's sleep can prevent a seizure from occurring the following day.

I would add that people with epilepsy should pay particular attention to getting enough rest and taking their antiepileptic medications at the appropriate time while traveling. When I was practicing in Charlotte, NC, it was not uncommon for patients to come to my office after a seizure at the airport. The stress of traveling, often accompanied by fatigue and missed antiepileptic medication, appeared to be a recipe for breakthrough seizures.

72. What about exercise?

Exercise provokes seizures in some patients, but this is uncommon. The potential benefits of physical fitness, improved mood, and increased socialization from exercise outweigh a risk of seizures in most patients. A child or adult should not be discouraged from exercising unless this activity clearly precipitates seizures. Regular exercise may actually improve seizure control.

73. Are there any modern alternative treatments for epilepsy?

VAGUS NERVE STIMULATOR

A device called the vagus nerve stimulator received Food and Drug Administration (FDA) approval in 1997 for the treatment of epilepsy (Question #180.) Since then, more than 40,000 people with intractable epilepsy have been treated with the vagus nerve stimulator worldwide. Similar in concept to a cardiac pacemaker, this device sends an electric shock to the vagus nerve in the neck at regular intervals. The vagus nerve transmits the electrical signal to the brain. These electrical impulses are believed to interfere with the process that allows epileptic seizures to develop.

Patients with many seizure types may benefit, including partial seizures, idiopathic generalized seizures, and patients with Lennox-Gastaut syndrome. The vagus nerve stimulator rarely results in complete seizure control. Consequently, before getting a vagus nerve stimulator, you should be evaluated at an epilepsy center to determine whether you might become seizure free with epilepsy surgery (Chapter 7). If you appear to be a good surgical candidate, you should seriously consider this option before getting a vagus nerve stimulator.

The most common side effects of the vagus nerve stimulator are cough, hoarseness, and throat pain, which result from stimulation of the vagus nerve in the neck. Unlike many seizure medications, the vagus nerve stimulator does not cause drowsiness. Consequently, it can be combined with antiepileptic medication therapy without an increase in typical medication side effects. Serious complications from the vagus nerve stimulator are rare.

The vagus nerve stimulator has recently received FDA approval for treatment of chronic or recurrent depression that doesn't respond to four or more antidepressant treatments. Because of the vagus nerve stimulator's beneficial effect on depression, it may be helpful for people who suffer from both epilepsy and depression.

You can get more information about the vagus nerve stimulator from a comprehensive epilepsy center (Appendix D) near you and at www.cyberonics.com.

TRANSCRANIAL MAGNETIC STIMULATOR

Transcranial magnetic stimulation is under investigation for the treatment of seizures and mood disorders and is now being evaluated in clinical trials (Question #180). This device delivers a magnetic pulse to the brain in the hopes of decreasing seizures or improving mood. However, transcranial magnetic stimulation may also cause seizures, and it is too early to tell whether this device will become a helpful therapy for people with epilepsy.

NEUROPACE RNS SYSTEM

Another new device under investigation is the NeuroPace RNS System, which detects a seizure when it occurs and sends an electrical stimulation to stop it. The stimulator is implanted in the brain (Question #180).

7

BRAIN SURGERY?

The "scary feelings" began when Barry was ten years old.
Sometimes confusion followed these strange sensations. A neurologist determined that the scary feelings were epileptic auras and
that the episodes of confusion were partial complex seizures. At first,
seizures occurred only once or twice a year. The scary feeling, which
was his aura, usually lasted about 30 seconds, giving him sufficient
warning and allowing him to pull off the side of the road if he was
driving. But at age 26, a seizure occurred without an aura and Barry had
a bad car accident. Luckily, he was not seriously injured and didn't hurt
anyone else. Frightened of what might have happened, Barry gave up his
driver's license.

Over the next few years, Barry's seizures increased. He relied on
his family, neighbors, and coworkers to get him to and from work. He
told me that he felt limited as a father because he couldn't drive his son
to school or sports events.

Barry worked hard to get his seizures under control. He took his
antiepileptic medication regularly, didn't drink alcohol, got enough
sleep, and tried to learn more about epilepsy. At a lecture I gave to an
epilepsy support group, he raised his hand and asked if I could help him.
We decided to work together.

After trying most of the traditional antiepileptic medications,
Barry participated in an investigational drug trial. His seizures improved
30 percent, but it was not enough to allow him to drive. He was afraid
of an operation on his brain, but it was his only real chance to become
seizure-free. Three years ago, Barry had a left temporal lobectomy.
Now, at age 41, he's driving a Jaguar.

74. What is epilepsy surgery?

There are several types of surgical operations designed to eliminate seizures. The most common one is anterior temporal lobectomy, in which the front part of the temporal lobe is removed.

Less commonly performed types of epilepsy surgery include removal of other lobes of the brain besides the temporal lobe, such as the frontal lobe or removal of several lobes (multilobar resection). In addition, other types of epilepsy surgery include corpus callosotomy, lesionectomy, localized neocortical resection, and multiple subpial transection.

75. Can epilepsy surgery be done in children?

Yes. Depending on the type of seizure and epilepsy syndrome, epilepsy surgery can be successfully performed in both children and adults. The youngest patient at our center to have a temporal lobectomy was seven years old. She is now seizure-free.

Once it is clear that antiepileptic medications are not going to be effective, there may be many advantages to epilepsy surgery early in life rather than later. Children seem to make faster and more complete neurological recovery after brain surgery. They are less likely to have heart or lung disease that can cause complications during an operation. In addition, once people have had disabling epilepsy for a long period of time, they often suffer severe psychological and social problems. Operating early on children may spare them these chronic problems and give them a better chance at living a healthy, productive life.

76. What is a callosotomy?

The two hemispheres of the brain are connected by white matter called the corpus callosum. In a corpus callosotomy, this structure is cut, decreasing the electrical communication between the two halves of the brain. In children with drop attacks, this operation can decrease the sudden falls.

Severing the corpus callosum can help control convulsions in patients who have multiple seizure foci and would not benefit from a temporal lobectomy or other types of surgery.

77. What is a hemispherectomy?

In some people, one hemisphere of the brain has been severely damaged and causes seizures and other neurological problems. A hemispherectomy removes or disconnects that part. Seizures, intellectual function, and social behavior may be surprisingly improved. In a recent study of hemispherectomy in 26 children with intractable epilepsy, more than 90% had significantly reduced seizures after surgery.

78. Is epilepsy surgery new?

No. Wilder Penfield, a famous American neurosurgeon who founded and designed the Montreal Neurological Institute, pioneered this surgery more than fifty years ago. By 1954, he had performed more than seven hundred and fifty operations. With improved physician training and technology, epilepsy surgery has become standardized and refined. To date, thousands of operations have been performed in epilepsy centers worldwide. The acceptance of epilepsy surgery for intractable epilepsy continues to grow.

79. Will I still have to take medication after the operation?

Most patients require antiepileptic medication in addition to epilepsy surgery to remain seizure-free. Often, the number of drugs and their dosages can be reduced. Some patients may no longer require any medication.

80. Who performs epilepsy surgery?

After a thorough evaluation by the epilepsy team, a neurosurgeon performs the operation with the assistance of an electrophysiologist (a brain wave specialist), an anesthesiologist, nurses, and other assistants.

81. Who is on the epilepsy team?

At a comprehensive epilepsy center, the team consists of an epilepsy coordinator, electroencephalograph technologists, a social worker, neuroscience nurses, neuropsychologists, neuropsychiatrists, neurologists, electrophysiologists, and neurosurgeons.

82. Who is a surgical candidate?

Candidates for surgery are patients whose seizures significantly decrease quality of life despite adequate trials of antiepileptic medication. Candidates for surgery should have an evaluation at a comprehensive epilepsy center to determine whether they are likely to benefit from epilepsy surgery.

83. Won't surgery result in a scar on my brain that could cause more seizures?

The excellent results with epilepsy surgery show that this is extremely unlikely to occur. We have never had a patient develop a new epilepsy focus as a result of seizure surgery.

84. How can I still be all right after having part of my brain removed?

Most people are understandably reluctant to lose any part of their body, particularly their brain! But epilepsy surgery removes damaged brain. Many people note no loss of function after surgery. (Barry is still working at his accounting job across the street from my office.) Some people even have intellectual improvement because the damaged part is no longer interfering with normal brain function.

85. Can the surgery make my seizures worse?

Approximately 10 to 15% of patients will have no improvement after seizure surgery, but it is very unlikely for seizures to get worse.

86. What is the chance I'll be seizure-free?

This varies for each patient, and you must discuss the expected outcome with your neurologist. Overall, temporal lobectomy eliminates seizures in about 60% of patients and at least another 25% are significantly improved. Certain patients with a well-defined seizure focus have a 90% chance of becoming seizure-free. After you receive a thorough preoperative evaluation, your neurologist will be able to tell you your chances of becoming seizure-free (Question #87).

87. What testing must be done before the operation?

Patients are admitted to the epilepsy monitoring unit for video/electroencephalographic (CCTV/EEG) localization of their seizure focus. Additionally, they require magnetic resonance imaging (MRI), a neuropsychological evaluation, and possibly a Wada (intracarotid amobarbital) test.

Some patients will have positron emission tomography (PET) and single photon emission computed tomography (SPECT) scans as well. One or more admissions to the hospital may be required, usually for a total of one to three weeks. The exact type of tests and duration of testing varies depending upon the patient's needs and also between epilepsy centers.

88. Can someone stay with me while I'm being monitored?

In our center, large chairs that convert into beds at night are provided in patient rooms. Family members and close friends become part of the epilepsy team. They are often the first to recognize a seizure when it begins and can notify the nursing staff.

89. What happens in an epilepsy monitoring unit?

Most epilepsy surgery is based on the principle that a single focus of epileptic activity causes the seizures. The purpose of monitoring is to locate that focus so that it can be surgically removed, leaving as much normal brain behind as possible.

Initially, electrodes are pasted or glued to your scalp. Tiny wires, called sphenoidal electrodes, may also be inserted through the skin in your cheeks.

If the seizure focus cannot be determined with scalp and sphenoidal electrodes, a neurosurgeon may need to place sterile electrodes inside your skull. Depending upon the clinical situation, different types of electrodes may be used. Two common types of intracranial electrodes are "strips," placed on the surface of the brain, or "depth," placed deep inside the brain.

90. Why do I have to see a neuropsychologist? I'm not crazy!

Living with epilepsy produces stress. People with epilepsy experience the stress of potential embarrassment and injury from unpredictable seizures, concerns over antiepileptic medication side effects, stigma, and education and employment difficulties. All of these stressors are good reasons to work with your doctor to try and control seizures medically or surgically.

In addition, being cured of epilepsy by an operation can also be stressful. Although epilepsy surgery may eliminate or decrease the frequency of seizures literally overnight, other changes such as getting a better education, a better job, and improving social relationships may be more difficult and take much longer. A neuropsychologist or psychiatrist helps people with epilepsy understand and cope with the many psychosocial issues of epilepsy.

Additionally, a neuropsychologist is trained to evaluate brain function. Extensive testing before the operation helps determine the site of the epileptic focus, as well as the chances of successful surgery. Postoperative testing evaluates whether any changes in thinking, memory, language, mood, or behavior have occurred.

All presurgical patients should be evaluated by a neuropsychologist.

91. What is a Wada test?

More than fifty years ago, Dr. Juhn Wada pioneered the use of intracarotid amobarbital injections at the Montreal Neurological Institute to assess language and memory in epilepsy surgery patients. The test is also known as the intracarotid amobarbital test because amobarbital is the drug traditionally used. During the Wada test, amobarbital or a comparable drug is injected first into a large artery on one side of the brain, then the other. This is done in the x-ray department by a neuroradiologist. Other drugs that may be used in place of amobarbital include etomidate, methohexital, or propofol.

The Wada test is done for two reasons. The first is to determine whether speech is located in the right or left temporal lobe.

The neurosurgeon needs this information in order to work around the speech center during the operation so that it is not damaged. The second purpose is to evaluate memory function. Because part of the memory center is removed during a temporal lobectomy, it is important to make sure the patient will not have noticeable memory loss after the operation. The Wada test determines whether the other temporal lobe works well enough to do the job alone. If the memory centers in both temporal lobes are damaged, the patient may not be able to have surgery.

92. What are depth electrodes?

Successful epileptic surgery requires precise localization of the brain region where the seizures begin. Sometimes the epileptic focus cannot be found using electrodes pasted on the scalp because they are too far away from the seizure focus. One option is to insert depth electrodes inside the brain, providing a much better chance of finding the origin of the seizures.

93. What is a grid?

A grid is a delicate array of electrodes placed on the surface of the brain by a neurosurgeon. Grids can be useful to localize the seizure focus when it is on the surface of the brain, the cerebral cortex. They are also used for speech mapping.

94. What is speech mapping?

In some patients, the epileptic focus is near the brain's speech center. If so, sometimes an electrophysiologist performs electrical stimulation of the brain to identify the exact location of the speech center. This map helps the neurosurgeon remove all of the epileptic tissue and preserve language function.

95. Will I be awake during the surgery?

Some neurosurgeons prefer to operate on the patient while awake so that speech and other neurological functions can be assessed. Local anesthesia is given and there is no pain. In our center, brain mapping is performed several days before surgery with the patient awake. The actual operation is done with the patient asleep.

96. How long does the surgery take?

A temporal lobectomy typically takes from four to six hours. After surgery, the patient goes to the intensive care unit for a day or two, then to a regular hospital room.

97. How long is the postoperative recovery period?

Most patients leave the hospital after a week. They are back to work in one to three months. Among patients who were unemployed prior to epilepsy surgery, approximately 25% find employment within two years of their operation. Patients who are seizure-free after surgery have the best chances of finding a job.

98. What kind of complications can I expect?

Significant medical complications are rare. At our center, two patients had strokes from which they made a near 100% recovery. Other problems can occur, such as language or memory difficulties. Some patients have psychological complications, experiencing changes in personality or mood or difficulty adjusting to life with few or no seizures. Part of the purpose of the extensive presurgical evaluation is to limit the possibility of medical or psychological side effects.

When people with epilepsy become seizure-free, opportunities that may never have been available to them may magically appear, such as the ability to drive, find a job, travel, and socialize with people who may not have been interested in them before. In addition, family members and friends may increase their demands on someone who is seizure-free, expecting them to contribute financially and in other ways. These sudden, dramatic changes in life can be overwhelming. Psychological counseling may be necessary to help the patient adjust to life without seizures.

99. How much does epilepsy surgery cost?

In addition to the expense of the surgery itself, anesthesia, and physician charges, there is the cost of the diagnostic evaluation including epilepsy monitoring, hospitalization, neuropsychological evaluation, and neuroimaging. Neuroimaging may include magnetic resonance imaging (MRI), positron emission tomography (PET), and single photon emission computed tomography (SPECT). Depending on the complexity of your case, costs range from $25,000 to more than $100,000.

100. Will my insurance cover it?

The extent of coverage varies with your individual policy. Speak with the epilepsy coordinator and your insurance representative before beginning the surgery evaluation to answer this question.

101. I want to get rid of my seizures. Can I have epilepsy surgery?

I do not encourage any of my patients to consider surgery until they have tried at least three or four antiepileptic medications and worked closely for a year or more with a neurologist experienced in seizure care. Additionally, you must be highly motivated.

An epilepsy surgery evaluation typically takes months of time and effort and is expensive. After all the information is obtained, an epilepsy team reviews the patient's history, neurological examination, neuropsychological results, electroencephalographs (EEGs), EEG and video monitoring results, and neuroimaging. After a thorough discussion of the findings, the team determines the likelihood of benefit from seizure surgery as well as the risks to that particular patient.

Although there are risks involved with brain surgery, living with intractable epilepsy has risks of its own. In addition to the socially disabling effects of seizures, some of my patients suffer repeated, painful injuries. In addition, there is a very low, but increased risk of death in people with epilepsy compared to the general population. This risk appears to be greatest in those with poorly controlled seizures.

At an office visit, I explain the team's recommendations. Then it is up to each patient to decide whether the time, trouble, risks, and expense are worth a chance at seizure control.

8

CAN I DRIVE?

Sam is fifteen years old and has partial complex seizures. He also has diabetes and takes insulin. Two years ago, he went thirteen months seizure-free, but then the seizures returned. Now he has a seizure once every few months. He has tried multiple antiepileptic medications without regaining complete control of his seizures. Sometimes Sam loses consciousness, and it's not clear whether he took too much insulin or had an epileptic seizure. He recently enrolled in a research study with a new antiepileptic drug in the hope of becoming seizure-free.

At his high school, Sam began classroom driver's education classes with the rest of his friends. He asked me when he would be able to start driving lessons in a car. When he learned that his state required a year of seizure freedom before he could apply for his driving license, he burst out crying. His father asked me when Sam would outgrow his seizures.

102. Why can't Sam drive?

There are two good reasons. The first is that his seizures remain uncontrolled. Sam has partial complex seizures, a type of seizure in which consciousness is altered. With each seizure, he becomes confused for several minutes. As a matter of public safety, anyone with uncontrolled partial complex seizures should not be driving an automobile or other moving vehicle like a tractor or lawnmower. People with other medical conditions such as alcoholism, cardiovascular disease, dementia or diabetes may also face limitation of their driving privileges.

The second reason is that Sam is having frequent insulin reactions and loses consciousness. He should not be driving until he learns to better regulate his diabetes, which will come with experience and more maturity.

103. Can anyone with seizures drive?

One of the major concerns of people with epilepsy is obtaining (or maintaining) their driver's license. Each state has different rules administered by their Department of Motor Vehicles (Appendix E). These regulations attempt to balance the need for the individual to drive against the risk of harm to the driver, passengers, and anyone else on the road should a seizure occur. These laws may change from year to year. Check with your local Department of Motor Vehicles regarding driving restrictions for people with epilepsy. People with uncontrolled epilepsy who drive may be breaking the law. People with epilepsy are not eligible for interstate commercial trucking licenses.

104. Wouldn't it be safe for Sam to drive when he grows out of his seizures?

Yes. However, Sam's magnetic resonance imaging (MRI) scan shows left temporal lobe atrophy, a structural abnormality that will not go away. He does not have a benign childhood epilepsy, such as benign Rolandic epilepsy, which he would outgrow. I have explained to Sam and his father that his type of epilepsy may be lifelong unless he responds to a new antiepileptic drug or possibly epilepsy surgery (Chapter 7). Although I encourage both of them to be optimistic, and I work very hard with Sam to control his seizures, it is counterproductive to base his future plans on wishful thinking.

105. Will Sam be able to drive if he goes a year seizure-free?

Even though legally he would be able to drive after one year in most states, given Sam's history of recurrent seizures,

I would personally like to see him seizure-free a little longer. It is important to be certain that his seizures are completely controlled before he gets behind the wheel. I would also like to be confident that he has learned to better manage his diabetes. For other patients, a seizure-free interval of as little as 3 months might be adequate. In one study, factors associated with a decreased risk of motor vehicle accidents in people with epilepsy were:

○ Seizure freedom for a year or more

○ Auras before every seizure

○ Few prior motor vehicle accidents not related to seizures

○ A change in antiepileptic drug treatment

When I make a recommendation regarding driving for a person with epilepsy, I take into account the local state regulations as well as the individual patient's type of epilepsy, adherence to therapy, past seizure frequency, medical conditions, and other factors.

106. What about people who only have seizures in their sleep?

A small percentage of people with epilepsy never have a seizure while awake. They may have one in the daytime while taking a nap, but otherwise only at night in their sleep. These patients may qualify for an exemption from the seizure-free period required by their state.

107. What about patients with other seizure types? Can they drive?

Yes. I have one patient who has a seizure every month, yet he is able to drive. He describes a warning in his head. This allows him to prepare for the rest of the seizure. Then his right arm feels as if it were blown up like a balloon, and it moves up and down. Afterwards it feels numb. Although inconvenient, these seizures do not cause any alteration of consciousness or significantly interfere with his driving and the safety of others.

Many other patients with partial simple seizures that cause minimal symptoms are able to drive. For example, these symptoms could include a twitch in the cheek or a tingling in an arm or leg. Generalized seizures and seizures with loss of awareness, of course, are not compatible with safe driving.

108. Are there any other circumstances in which a patient with uncontrolled seizures can drive?

Yes. Some patients have prolonged auras. They can sense a seizure coming, either by a "funny feeling," a strong odor, or other warning. If the aura is long enough, they will have time to drive a car to the side of the road. The Department of Motor Vehicles may allow exemptions for patients whose seizures are always associated with auras.

109. What if my seizures are not controlled and I need to drive to work?

In the United States, public transportation is often lacking, and driving can be essential to a successful work and social life. Unfortunately, the need for transportation does not give one the privilege to drive a car. Carpooling may be a practical and cost-effective option. One of my patients, now seizure-free after a temporal lobectomy, shuttles two epilepsy patients from her hometown to their regular office visits with me.

You may find some solutions to transportation problems by talking with other people who have epilepsy at local support group meetings or by contacting your Epilepsy Foundation state affiliate (Appendix C).

110. Will my doctor report me if I keep having seizures and continue to drive?

In most states, it is not the physician's legal obligation to notify the Department of Motor Vehicles when patients are having seizures. However, your physician may do this if it appears that you are driving and putting yourself and others at unacceptable risk or if required by your state (Appendix E).

The American Academy of Neurology recently (2007) published a position statement recommending that physician reporting of individuals with uncontrolled seizures should be optional.* Mandatory reporting of individuals with uncontrolled seizures violates the patient's privacy and may adversely affect the patient-doctor relationship. The Academy advises physicians to discuss local driving laws with their patients. Ideally, you should be comfortable telling your doctor everything about your seizures without fear that you will be reported. Remember, your doctor's primary role is to help you manage your seizures and live as healthy and productive a life as possible.

111. How can I convince my doctor to let me drive?

It is not your doctor you have to persuade. It is the Department of Motor Vehicles—they make the rules. To get a driver's license, make your best effort to work with your doctor to eliminate your seizures. That means taking your antiepileptic medication as directed, filling in your seizure calendar, keeping appointments, and being willing to consider sophisticated therapy, such as epilepsy surgery (Chapter 7), the vagus nerve stimulator (Question #73), or an investigational antiepileptic drug (Chapter 14).

---

*Bacon D, Fisher RS, Morris JC, et al. American Academy of Neurology position statement on physician reporting of medical conditions that may affect driving competence. Neurology 2007;68:1174-1177.

If you think you have been unjustly denied a driver's license, ask your doctor for his opinion. If he agrees, consider appealing the decision. Most states permit an appeal. Whether you can drive or not is a safety issue, a decision that boils down to common sense.

9

SEIZURES AND WORK

Treatment with phenytoin (Dilantin®) and carbamazepine
(Tegretol®) didn't stop Bob's seizures. After several years of
trial and error with different antiepileptic drugs, we finally succeeded
with a combination of divalproex sodium (Depakote®), gabapentin
(Neurontin®), and acetazolamide (Diamox®). Bob also made lifestyle
changes (gave up drugs and alcohol) and improved his adherence to
antiepileptic medication.

For the past year, Bob has been seizure-free and gainfully employed.
Trained as an aircraft engineer, he repairs Teflon strips on propeller
blades using adhesives, chemicals, and glues.

Last month, I received a letter from his employer who observed
that Bob had "poor memory for details, increased scrap rate, difficulty
following instructions, and multiple mistakes." The employer asked for
my advice.

112. Can people with epilepsy work?

A large number of people with epilepsy hold successful
careers and work as administrators, business owners, clerks and
salespeople, nurses, technicians, and at other jobs. On the other
hand, many do not work. For people with epilepsy, unemployment is greater than twice the national average, with more than
25% of individuals with epilepsy unemployed. A chart review of
306 of my patients with well-documented epilepsy revealed that
18% of them received disability compensation.

113. Why can't people with epilepsy work?

The most frequent problem I see is that seizures interfere with the job. One of my patients worked for the local utility company maintaining power lines. He pruned trees with a chain saw while standing in a bucket supported two stories above the street by a crane. When he developed epilepsy, it was impractical for him to continue working at this hazardous job.

In North Carolina, many of my patients worked in textile mills. When they developed epilepsy, it became unsafe for them to work with the fast moving, dangerous machinery.

Similarly, people who drive for a living, whether chauffeuring a taxi or bus, delivering the mail, or going on regional sales calls are unable to continue their jobs when they develop uncontrolled seizures.

In situations like these, it is reasonable to approach your employer to see whether there is another job at the same business that a person with uncontrolled seizures could perform safely, such as secretarial work or other "desk job." This might be a temporary position until your seizures come under control and you can resume your previous job.

114. What about shift work?

Many people with epilepsy have more seizures when they are sleep deprived. To control your seizures, it is best to try and keep a regular schedule. Take your antiepileptic medication at the same time every day. Get as much sleep as you need. Try and avoid jobs where you must keep changing your schedule. If your job requires changing shifts, discuss this with your supervisor and see if an exception can be made for you, which could be considered a "reasonable accommodation" for a person with epilepsy under the Americans with Disabilities Act (Question #119). If you have to change shifts, make sure you don't miss your antiepileptic medication and get enough sleep before coming to work. Avoid driving and other potentially hazardous activities until you are well adjusted to the new schedule.

115. I know someone with epilepsy who doesn't have seizures any more, but she still can't get a job. Why is that?

In some cases, other disabilities associated with epilepsy limit employment. For example, approximately 9% of children with epilepsy have mental retardation. This additional problem limits their educability and job opportunities in the future.

One of my patients didn't develop epilepsy until he was twenty years old, but he had never worked. He said it was because of his birth defect, a type of cerebral palsy. He has slurred speech and a mild paralysis of his right side with a clumsy right hand. These disabilities kept him from working, not the epilepsy.

Sometimes sedative side effects from antiepileptic medication interfere with job performance. Often these side effects can be decreased by dose adjustments, a switch to another antiepileptic medication, or decreasing the number of antiepileptic drugs.

It is also possible that discrimination because of epilepsy can limit job opportunities. However, most complaints of discrimination in the workplace by people with epilepsy are not related to job hiring, but rather address issues of disciplinary action, harassment, promotion, and termination, which occur after hiring.

116. How can I keep discrimination from preventing me from getting a job?

Discrimination in employment is outlawed by the Americans with Disabilities Act of 1990, Public Law 101-336. This law supplements the Rehabilitation Act of 1973, which prohibits discrimination by federal contractors, federal agencies, or recipients of federal financial assistance. These laws prevent discrimination in employment on the basis of prejudice and ignorance.

The Americans with Disabilities Act applies to private businesses, state and local governments, employment agencies, labor unions, and joint labor-management committees with more than 15 employees. Just as it is illegal to discriminate on the basis of race or sex, this law makes it illegal to discriminate on the basis of epilepsy. However, the person applying for the job must be willing and able to do the work.

117. What if they ask for a drug test? Do I have to take it?

Yes. Drug tests are designed to screen for drug abuse and may be required before you begin employment. However, the presence of antiepileptic medication in your urine cannot be used to disqualify you for the job.

118. What about a medical examination?

An employer is not permitted to ask health-related questions during an interview or on a job application. A medical history and examination can only be required after a job offer is made. It is illegal for an employer to use the fact that you have epilepsy to disqualify you.

119. How does the Americans with Disabilities Act protect me?

Another feature of the Americans with Disabilities Act is the "reasonable accommodation" provision. This language requires the employer to make changes in the work environment or job description if the applicant can otherwise fulfill all the "essential functions" of employment. My patient, Karen, was in her early forties and had a successful banking job. She worked in

Valley Cottage Free Library

User ID: 22841000230848

Title: The essential Caribbean cookbook :
50 classic rec
Item ID: 32841000673281
Date due: 6/25/2012,23:59

Title: Building a web site for dummies
Item ID: 32841009403435
Date due: 6/25/2012,23:59

Title: Ageless with Kathy Smith. Staying s
trong [DVD]
Item ID: 32841009451971
Date due: 6/10/2012,23:59

Title: Sams teach yourself WordPress in 10
 minutes
Item ID: 32841009315481
Date due: 6/25/2012,23:59

Title: Epilepsy : 199 answers : a doctor r
esponds to his
Item ID: 32841009235036
Date due: 6/25/2012,23:59

Title: Colombiana [DVD]
Item ID: 32841009520403
Date due: 5/30/2012,23:59

Questions? Call 845-268-7700
www.vclib.org

administration, where her monthly partial complex seizures were not a major problem. She usually would have a brief warning and sit down at her desk or go to the ladies room until the seizure was over. She did her work well and was advancing in management.

Last year, the bank acquired its first out-of-town branch office, which required an inspection every three months. Branch supervision was part of Karen's responsibility. Even though she couldn't drive, she had never had a problem with this aspect of her job as she could take a cab to all the local branches. In order to inspect this new rural acquisition, she would have to take a short flight and then rent a car. Because of her uncontrolled seizures, traveling alone by plane and renting a car presented major obstacles.

Although it was her responsibility, this particular branch inspection could be performed by one of her colleagues. It was also a very small part of her job, not an "essential function." Consequently, when Karen asked her boss to relieve her of this obligation, the only aspect of her job she could not do, she was protected by the Americans with Disabilities Act. It was possible for her boss to make a "reasonable accommodation" by assigning this trip to someone else and letting Karen continue doing her good work at the home office. More information on "reasonable accommodation" may be found in the Technical Assistance Manual of the Americans with Disabilities Act on the Job Accommodation Networks website: www.jan.wvu.edu/links/ADAtam1.html or by calling (800) 514-0301.

120. Does the Americans with Disabilities Act keep me from getting fired?

Jack worked at a nature museum. Initially, his seizures were controlled, but as he got older, his epilepsy became more severe. Despite increasing doses of antiepileptic medication, he began having seizures at work and would become confused and wander off.

Jack's primary job was feeding the animals and cleaning their cages. Some of the animals, such as raccoons and foxes, were potentially dangerous. One day, while bringing breakfast to a valuable arctic fox, Jack had a seizure and left the cage open. When his mind cleared and he realized what had happened, he searched all over the museum, but he couldn't find the fox.

The next day, the animal was found dead on a nearby highway. Jack was fired when the details of the incident became clear to his employer.

Jack was furious over losing his job and contacted a lawyer. He said he wanted to sue because of discrimination. The attorney advised Jack that the law did not protect him in this case. He was not being discriminated against because he had epilepsy. He was let go because his uncontrolled seizures did not allow him to do his job properly or safely.

121. Who should I contact if I have a concern about discrimination?

Call your state affiliate (Appendix C) or the national office of the Epilepsy Foundation (800) 332-1000. They will be able to provide you with more information and direct you to the proper legal resources.

122. Who at work should I tell?

If it is likely that you will have a seizure at work, you should inform your supervisor and close coworkers. Otherwise, after your first seizure on the job, you will probably get whisked off to the emergency room. Your coworkers will be best prepared to help you if they are forewarned.

When you discuss your epilepsy, you will have an opportunity to educate your coworkers about appropriate first aid. Share the first aid information in Appendix J with them. You can also provide guidelines regarding when to call an ambulance. If your supervisor wants more information, you can suggest that he call your doctor, a local epilepsy center, the Epilepsy Foundation (or read this book!).

You may wish to create an "Action Plan" that includes your emergency contact numbers and a plan of action should you have a seizure. A form for this purpose is provided by the Job Accommodation Network (JAN) as a service of the US Department of Labor Office of Disability Employment Policy (Appendix L). This document may include information such as warning signs that you are going to have a seizure, instructions on first aid and when to call an ambulance, and other information that you would want your employer and colleagues to know should you have a seizure in the workplace. Complete this form and review it with your employer. This document is kept at work in your confidential medical file.

123. Should I wear a MedicAlert bracelet?

This is a personal decision. Some people are private about their seizures. Others, particularly those with frequent seizures, have learned that communication about their disorder can benefit them. For example, if a police officer finds you confused in a parking lot late Saturday night, he is likely to consider epilepsy rather than alcohol intoxication when he sees a MedicAlert bracelet.

Some people with epilepsy prefer to wear a MedicAlert necklace, as this is more discreet, but would be found by health professionals or others in an emergency. Ask your doctor for his opinion.

124. What if I can't find a job?

Finding the right job is difficult for everyone, whether they have epilepsy or not. Frequent seizures increase the likelihood of unemployment. Work with your doctor to control your seizures. A positive attitude toward work can help. A recent survey of more than 250 people attending an epilepsy center in Florida revealed that those who perceived the importance of work for personal reasons, had decreased fears of workplace discrimination, and had a higher annual family income were more likely to be employed.

If you continue to have difficulty finding a job, look to others who may be able to help you. If you are in school, career counselors are available. If you have finished school, ask your doctor for a referral to a social worker or vocational rehabilitation.

125. What is the Employment Signature Program?

Over the years, various programs have been in place to facilitate employment for people with epilepsy. These include TAPS (Training Applicants for Placement Success), which was funded by the US Department of Labor, and JobTech, which was developed by the Epilepsy Foundation and sponsored by the US Department of Labor and the US Social Security Administration.

The Epilepsy Foundation has developed a new Employment Signature Program, which features a manual of strategies and resources that may be used locally and in conjunction with the national Epilepsy Foundation office to increase employment of people with epilepsy. The manual includes an Employer Awareness Program to educate potential employers about the issues regarding hiring people with epilepsy. This manual is scheduled for publication in 2007.

126. My seizures are perfectly controlled. Are there any jobs I still can't qualify for?

The federal Department of Transportation prohibits anyone with a history of seizures from obtaining a federal commercial driver's license. Similarly, the Federal Aviation Administration disqualifies anyone with a history of epilepsy from becoming a commercial pilot.There are no other legal restrictions that prevent people with controlled seizures from working.

127. What about the armed forces?

Enlistment in one of the branches of the armed forces is possible if you are seizure-free without medications for at least five years and have a normal electroencephalogram.

128. What happened to Bob? Did his work performance improve?

I made sure his antiepileptic drug levels weren't toxic, and Bob tried without success to boost the quality of his work. I wrote a letter on his behalf, but Bob lost his job. Even though he wasn't having seizures, he was not able to meet the required standards of his position. Now he works for another company as a fluid hydraulics mechanic and is doing fine.

10

WOMEN AND EPILEPSY

> J ill was twenty-two years old and four months pregnant when we met at the obstetrics clinic two years ago. It was the first time she had seen a neurologist since she was a teenager. Even though she had not had a seizure in years, she was still taking two epilepsy medications, phenytoin (Dilantin®) and phenobarbital. Her pregnancy was going well, and she was reluctant to decrease her antiepileptic medications for fear of a seizure. After she delivered (luckily, a healthy baby), I ordered a sleep-deprived electroencephalogram (EEG) and magnetic resonance imaging (MRI) scan. Since both studies were normal, we decided to decrease one antiepileptic medication with the intention of stopping it if she continued seizure-free. After a longer period of observation, we could consider stopping the second drug as well.
>
> Although Jill insisted she had no plans for another baby, she reluctantly agreed to take prenatal vitamins and folate. Over a few months, we gradually decreased the dose of phenobarbital and discontinued it. She had her phenytoin level checked regularly, and we kept it in the low therapeutic range. Last month she appeared in the obstetrics clinic again, embarrassed but with a smile on her face. She was pregnant again! We both felt reassured that we had done everything we could to ensure a healthy baby.

129. Why do I have seizures only around the time of my period?

Some women have seizures related to their monthly cycle. This is called catamenial epilepsy, which appears related to estrogen and progesterone fluctuations during the menstrual cycle. Estrogen has proconvulsant effects and progesterone anticonvulsant effects;

changes in the concentrations of these hormones may affect seizure control. Use your seizure calendar to see whether your seizures only occur with your monthly period. If you have catamenial epilepsy, your doctor may want to prescribe acetazolamide (Diamox®), hormonal therapy, or other treatment in addition to your antiepileptic drugs. At present, there is no Food and Drug Administration (FDA)-approved therapy specific for catamenial epilepsy.

130. Will taking birth control pills cause me to have more seizures?

In general, oral contraceptives do not affect the blood levels of antiepileptic drugs and should not affect seizure control. An exception to this rule is the blood level of lamotrigine, which may decrease when taken with oral contraceptives. Breakthrough seizures may result. Conversely, when the oral contraceptives are stopped, lamotrigine levels will increase, possibly resulting in side effects. If you are taking birth control pills and lamotrigine, discuss the management of your drug level with your doctor.

131. Will antiepileptic drugs affect the efficacy of the birth control pill?

Because oral contraceptives and many antiepileptic drugs are metabolized by the liver, there is the possibility that one may affect the metabolism of the other. Certain antiepileptic medications, including carbamazepine (Tegretol®), oxcarbazepine (Trileptal®), phenobarbital, phenytoin (Dilantin®), primidone (Mysoline®), and topiramate (Topamax®) can increase the metabolism of the birth control pill and render it less effective, which means that pregnancy may occur. Lamotrigine (Lamictal®) may also affect the metabolism of the birth control pill, but whether this is clinically significant is not yet certain. If you are taking one of these antiepileptic medications, you must discuss this issue with your neurologist and obstetrician to see if you need a stronger dosage of the birth control pill or a different form of contraception.

Divalproex sodium (Depakote®), gabapentin (Neurontin®), ethosuximide (Zarontin®), levetiracetam (Keppra®), pregabalin (Lyrica®), and zonisamide (Zonegran®) do not affect the birth control pill.

132. What about levonorgestrel implants (Norplant®) or medroxyprogesterone (Depo-Provera®)?

Because these are also hormonal therapies, the same cautions given for the birth control pill apply. One of my patients became pregnant while taking carbamazepine (Tegretol®) and using the levonorgestrel implant. She wasn't ready for another child and the pregnancy caused a great deal of stress.

133. What is the best medication for treating seizures in pregnancy?

Although you may hear differently, it is now generally agreed that the best choice of epilepsy medication in pregnancy is the drug that eliminates the most seizures with the fewest side effects. You and your neurologist must choose the antiepileptic drug that is best for you.

134. How will pregnancy affect my seizure frequency?

Seizure frequency may increase during pregnancy. Part of the reason for this increase is that many women stop their epilepsy medications. This is usually *not* the best thing to do. Seizures may also occur because pregnancy can cause poor absorption of medication and an increase in antiepileptic drug metabolism, both of which result in lower drug levels. In order to have the best control of seizures during pregnancy, it is essential to visit both your obstetrician and neurologist regularly. Because of the dramatic changes in your body, you will need to have drug levels measured more frequently. Your dosage may need to be increased, particularly during the third trimester, and then decreased promptly after delivery. This last bit of advice is often forgotten because the woman goes home from the hospital and is busy with her new baby. But now that the pregnancy is over, antiepileptic drug levels may rise and cause symptoms of toxicity. Make sure you follow up with your neurologist a couple weeks after delivery to check on your antiepileptic drug doses and blood levels.

Another cause of increased seizures is lack of sleep. To avoid seizures, you must make a special effort to get enough rest. Because it is so important to get adequate rest, try and get help with your new baby.

135. Should I discontinue my epilepsy medications if I become pregnant?

Approximately one-third of people with epilepsy are women of childbearing age, so this is an important question. Although antiepileptic medications may cause birth defects, they usually do not. The risk of birth defects in children to women with epilepsy is about 6%. That means there is a 94% chance there will be no birth defects.

The most serious birth defects occur early in pregnancy, before you even know you're pregnant. That is why stopping your antiepileptic medication will probably increase your seizures and not help your baby very much.

It is not clear which antiepileptic drug has the lowest risk for birth defects and developmental problems. Based on new data from the pregnancy registries, divalproex sodium (Depakote®)

may contribute to congenital malformations and cognitive problems in infants more than some of the other antiepileptic drugs.

However, regardless of which antiepileptic drug you are taking, you should not discontinue it until you have consulted your physician. The risk of harm to you and your baby from uncontrolled seizures may be higher than the risk to your baby from antiepileptic medication.

If you are taking antiepileptic medication, you may receive educational materials and participate in the Antiepileptic Drug Pregnancy Registry by calling 1-888-233-2334 (www.aedpregnancyregistry.org). Participation in the pregnancy registry is very important if we are to learn more about the effects of antiepileptic drugs on children born to women with epilepsy.

136. Is there a way to check for birth defects?

Yes. One blood test is called alpha-fetoprotein, which you should get at approximately 18 weeks, particularly if you are taking carbamazepine (Tegretol®) or divalproex sodium (Depakote®). It is also important to get an ultrasound at this time. These tests are another reason why it is important to have frequent visits with your obstetrician during your pregnancy.

137. I am taking three anticonvulsants. Is this worse than taking just one?

Yes. Planning your pregnancy with your doctor is an excellent opportunity to reevaluate the appropriateness of your antiepileptic medication. If your seizures are controlled, perhaps two medications would be sufficient. (Jill was able to do just fine on one.) Fewer drugs would lower the danger to your baby and decrease the likelihood that you will have side effects. You can work with your neurologist to adjust your antiepileptic medications so that you are taking the least number of drugs at the lowest dosages necessary to control your seizures.

138. What can I do to make sure I have a healthy baby?

Plan your pregnancy! That way you can begin taking prenatal vitamins and folic acid, make sure you eat nutritious foods, get enough sleep, and avoid alcohol, drugs, and cigarettes.

139. Are there any special vitamins I should take?

Yes. Before you become pregnant, you should take prenatal vitamins. If you are a sexually active woman of childbearing age, you should at the very least take a multivitamin every day, even if you are not planning to become pregnant. Many doctors also prescribe folic acid (1 mg to 4 mg/day), which may help prevent birth defects of the brain and spinal cord. At about 36 to 38 weeks, your doctor may also prescribe vitamin K, which may help prevent bleeding in the baby at the time of delivery.

140. Can seizures occur during delivery?

Yes, but only 1 to 2% of women with epilepsy have a convulsion during labor and delivery. This is a time of high stress, antiepileptic medications may have been missed, and sleep deprivation is likely. But seizures can be easily treated in the delivery room with intravenous medication such as diazepam (Valium®) or lorazepam (Ativan®). When you are admitted to the hospital in labor, make sure you bring your antiepileptic medication with you and tell the admitting physician (who may not be your regular doctor) about your epilepsy. In the hospital, your blood level of antiepileptic medication can be checked and additional medication given by mouth or intravenously if needed.

141. Can I breast-feed?

Epilepsy medication appears in the breast milk to some degree but usually does not affect the infant. The amount varies depending upon the particular epilepsy drug. Phenobarbital and primidone (Mysoline®) in breast milk can cause drowsiness in the baby and poor sucking. If this happens, you will have to bottle-feed. Otherwise, breast-feeding should not be a problem.

142. Will my seizures interfere with taking care of the baby?

If you have frequent partial complex or grand mal seizures, it may be unsafe for you to be the sole caretaker of an infant. There are some things you can do to lower the risks. When changing the baby, for example, do it on the floor rather than on a high table. Do not bathe the baby yourself. Try to find someone to help you with child care so that you do not become overtired.

Some women with frequent seizures cannot safely take care of a baby. You and your doctor should make this important decision together.

11

MY CHILD WITH EPILEPSY

> Jessica is a five-year-old girl I saw in the emergency room for her first seizure. She and her grandmother sleep in the same bed. Her grandmother told me that Jessica began "jerking and gasping" at five o'clock in the morning. She was unresponsive and staring, and the jerking lasted about ten minutes. Jessica had been coughing a little for the past few days, but had no fever. After the convulsion, her right side seemed weak for a few minutes.
>
> When I examined her, she had a low-grade temperature and slight wheezes in both lungs. Her strength had returned to normal. Jessica's computed axial tomography (CAT or CT) scan was unremarkable. Her electroencephalogram (EEG) revealed large epileptic spikes on the left side of her brain.
>
> I was able to reassure her distressed grandmother that Jessica had a benign focal epilepsy of childhood, Rolandic epilepsy, which she would outgrow. The seizure had probably been triggered by her bronchitis. Because the convulsion was so upsetting and prolonged, we decided to treat Jessica with antiepileptic medication until she no longer needed it.

143. Will my child grow out of her seizures?

Your neurologist can help you with prognosis by diagnosing the particular epileptic syndrome. The history, physical examination, brain imaging with computed axial tomography (CAT or CT) or magnetic resonance imaging (MRI), and particularly the electroencephalogram (EEG) all help your doctor arrive at an accurate classification of your child's epilepsy.

For example, if your child has Rolandic epilepsy, also known as benign epilepsy with centrotemporal spikes (BECTS), the most common type of childhood epilepsy, she will likely outgrow it during adolescence. On the other hand, if she has Lennox-Gastaut syndrome, she probably will not.

Although epilepsy can rarely be cured, much can be gained by obtaining an accurate diagnosis. This helps guide treatment and molds expectations for the future. (Had Jessica not been evaluated in the emergency room, her grandmother would have worried needlessly that Jessica would suffer seizures all her life.)

144. What is a febrile seizure?

Small children can have convulsions related to a high fever. Febrile seizures are common, occurring in 4% of children. When a first seizure occurs with fever, the child should be evaluated by a physician. A respiratory infection or gastroenteritis often causes the elevated temperature. If the seizure is prolonged, anticonvulsants will be needed, the body has to be cooled, and the underlying cause of the fever must be treated. Most doctors do not prescribe daily anticonvulsants after a first febrile seizure. If one child has febrile seizures, the risk of other siblings developing febrile seizures is approximately 8%.

Children outgrow febrile seizures by the age of five or six years. The vast majority do **not** go on to develop epilepsy. Risk factors for epilepsy are a preexisting neurological abnormality, onset of febrile seizures before one year of age, multiple or prolonged febrile seizures, and a family history of epilepsy. If your child has none of these risk factors, the likelihood of epilepsy is only about 1%.

145. Why can't they find a cause for the seizure? They told me all her tests are normal!

In more than 50% of children with epilepsy, no brain tumor, cyst, malformation, or "scar" explains the occurrence of a seizure. However, an intermittent electrical malfunction in the child's brain is responsible. Although the electroencephalogram (EEG) can be normal between seizures, the abnormal brain waves will usually be seen if a seizure occurs during an EEG.

When all the tests are normal and no cause is found, this is a good sign. These children's seizures tend to be more easily controlled.

146. Do seizures cause brain damage?

Children with absence, or petit mal, seizures can have many spells without apparent ill effects. After a staring spell, they can pick up where they left off in a conversation. Their electroencephalogram (EEG) returns to normal immediately.

People with partial complex or generalized seizures, however, do not return to normal right away. The postictal period immediately after a seizure is characterized by confusion and fatigue. The EEG often slows down after a seizure, supporting the concept that the brain has not fully recovered.

We do know that brain injury can occur when seizures last longer than 30 minutes, a condition termed status epilepticus (Question #16). Two of my adult patients had persistent memory loss after episodes of status epilepticus.

Whether brief seizures cause brain injury is unknown. Much research is currently focused on answering this question. Many of my patients with intractable temporal lobe epilepsy complain of memory difficulties. Whether this problem stems from their numerous seizures or the underlying cause of the epilepsy remains unclear.

It does appear prudent to control seizures when possible. Even though antiepileptic medications have potential side effects, they are usually a better choice than recurrent seizures.

147. What is the ketogenic diet?

Diet treatments for epilepsy have been prescribed for epilepsy since the time of Hippocrates. The diet that has been studied the longest and with the most research substantiating its effectiveness is the ketogenic diet. The ketogenic diet is usually prescribed for children who have not responded to treatment with antiepileptic medications.

Pioneered more than eighty-five years ago, the ketogenic diet is low in carbohydrate, has adequate protein, but is extremely high in fat. The diet contains up to five times more fat than protein and carbohydrates combined. It is what most adults would consider a very unhealthy diet. However, because of the slight calorie restriction, children do not gain excess weight. Fluids may also be restricted. In order to insure adequate nutrition, multivitamins, calcium, vitamin D, and other supplements may be given.

Because of its complexity, the ketogenic diet can only be followed under a neurologist's supervision with the assistance of a dietitian. The diet usually begins with a brief hospital admission for one to two days of fasting and meal preparation training. Many epilepsy centers are no longer fasting children, although the diet may work quicker if begun with a fast. The diet must be followed exactly. Each food portion is carefully weighed on a scale, and the entire meal must be eaten.

Exactly how the ketogenic diet controls seizures is largely unknown and remains a question under active investigation. We do know that the fat in the diet causes molecules called ketone bodies to accumulate, which may play a role in decreasing seizure frequency. To make sure that the appropriate amount of ketone bodies is being produced by the diet, they may be easily measured at home or in the clinic with a urine dipstick.

When the ketogenic diet is carefully followed, about 10 to 15% of children become seizure-free, and another 30% have their seizure frequency dramatically reduced. If the diet is going to be effective, seizure frequency usually decreases within a month. After two years of successful seizure control, the diet may be discontinued without return of seizures in about one in five patients. If seizures are not completely eliminated, parents may still choose to keep their children on the ketogenic diet, sometimes for many years.

The ketogenic diet does not work in every child. It is not yet clear why the diet works in some children but not in others. Children who are tube fed and those with infantile spasms or tuberous sclerosis often do well. More research on the mechanisms of action of the ketogenic diet as well as identifying children who are likely to respond is ongoing.

Carrying out this diet requires a strong parental commitment and your child's daily cooperation. About one in six children will not tolerate the diet. Stomach upset is common, with symptoms such as nausea, vomiting, diarrhea, or constipation. Other complications may include acidosis, bone fractures, elevated cholesterol, kidney stones, and stunted growth. If you are interested in trying the diet, discuss the potential benefits and risks with your pediatric neurologist. Antiepileptic drugs are usually continued while on the diet, at least for the first month. Although the diet is not a medication, it is a sophisticated treatment. You may need to go to a comprehensive epilepsy center to find a dietitian familiar with this program. After starting the diet, your child will have periodic medical checks, including blood tests, to monitor for possible complications.

If you wish to learn more about the ketogenic diet, an excellent book has been written for parents, dietitians, and physicians that should answer your questions. *The Ketogenic Diet, A Treatment for Children and Others with Epilepsy*, Fourth Edition, John M. Freeman, MD, Eric H. Kossoff, MD, Jennifer B. Freeman, Millicent T. Kelly, RD, LD, can be obtained from Demos Medical Publishing, 386 Park Avenue South, New York, NY, 10016, (800) 532-8663 (www.demosmedpub.com).

Another diet that restricts carbohydrates, but is easier to follow and may be better tolerated, is the modified Atkins diet. The modified Atkins diet allows unlimited calories, fat, protein, and fluids and was created by a group of pediatric neurologists at Johns Hopkins Medical Center in 2002. Early studies have shown promise for the modified Atkins diet to decrease seizure frequency. There is no need for a hospital admission or preparatory fast. Ketosis, created by the high-fat and low-carbohydrate diet, does not seem to be as important in controlling the seizures. Stomach problems, increased cholesterol, weight loss, and other side effects may also occur. In some patients, it may be possible to substitute a modified Atkins diet for the more demanding ketogenic diet. The modified Atkins diet may also be effective in adults with intractable seizures.

Both the ketogenic diet and the modified Atkins diet should be carried out under the supervision of your neurologist with the assistance of a trained dietician.

148. Are epilepsy and attention deficit hyperactivity disorder (ADHD) related?

Epilepsy affects approximately 1% of children, while ADHD affects 3 to 5%. Since these disorders are relatively common, some children have both. Most children with ADHD do not have epilepsy. If there is any question about the diagnosis, bring your child to see a pediatric neurologist who will take a detailed history, examine your child, and order an electroencephalogram (EEG).

However, many children with epilepsy may have symptoms consistent with ADHD. Problems paying attention and hyperactivity may result from epileptic activity between seizures (interictal), the seizures themselves (ictal), or brain dysfunction during the recovery period after seizures (postictal). Antiepileptic drugs may also contribute. In addition, it may be that the underlying cause of the epilepsy, such as a birth defect or brain injury, is also responsible for the symptoms of ADHD. ADHD symptoms affect one-third or more of children with epilepsy and are associated with decreased school performance and decreased quality of life.

Both behavioral and medication treatment are available for ADHD. Sometimes these problems may not be fully addressed in your visit with the neurologist because the focus is more on treating the epilepsy. If you suspect symptoms of ADHD in your child with epilepsy, discuss these concerns with your pediatric neurologist who can take steps to make a formal diagnosis and treatment plan.

149. Can video games cause seizures?

Less than 15% of people with epilepsy have seizures (called photosensitive epilepsy) in response to flashing lights. Children and adults with this type of seizure disorder need to avoid strobe lights, flickering television screens, and video games.

Sometimes children have their first seizure triggered by a video game, making it appear that the game caused their epilepsy. This is not the case. Children *without* epilepsy do not have seizures from video games.

Most children with epilepsy are not photosensitive. Before prohibiting your child from playing video games and watching television, ask your neurologist whether flashing lights present a risk. Photosensitive epilepsy can be easily diagnosed during testing with flashing lights and an electroencephalogram (EEG). See Question #20 for more information.

150. Can my child participate in sports?

One of the biggest dangers of epilepsy in children is the overprotectiveness it fosters in parents. To develop normally, children need to face many challenges, academic, athletic, and social, among others. To have a full life, they need to test their limits (and probably yours!).

Children with frequent seizures should not swim alone, horseback ride, rock climb, high dive, do gymnastics above the ground on the balance beam and rings, or participate in other sports in which a sudden alteration of consciousness could result in serious injury. Baseball, soccer, football, tennis, volleyball, and playground sports are safer. Children with less frequent seizures can participate in most sports. Exercise rarely causes seizures.

There is always the possibility of injury when participating in sports, even for a child without epilepsy. As a parent, you will have to weigh the risk of injury against the risk of depriving your child of an important facet of life. If your child rides a bicycle, a helmet is a good precaution, as it is for all children. While boating, every child should wear a life jacket, whether they have epilepsy or not. In order to decide which sports are appropriate for your child, discuss safety concerns with your child, his teacher, coach, and physician. An epilepsy summer camp may be a good environment for your child to learn and participate in sports under supervision (Appendix F).

151. I want my child to know he isn't the only one with epilepsy. What can I do?

A local support group where your child can meet other children with seizures may be helpful. The Epilepsy Foundation sponsors a School Alert program to provide epilepsy education. An educational puppet show, *Kids on the Block*, is available for children (www.kotb.com/). Contact the Epilepsy Foundation to see whether a program can be performed in your child's classroom. Knowledge of epilepsy can replace fear and provide a more supportive classroom environment for your child. Online communities such as www.epilepsy.com provide quality medical information and an opportunity to share personal experiences with epilepsy. Epilepsy.com has a special section for kids.

Over thirty summer camps are designed for children with epilepsy (Appendix F). Some are free of charge or scholarships may be available through the local affiliate. These camps provide an exposure to sports under supervision as well as an opportunity to interact with peers. Some camp counselors may have epilepsy as well and can serve as mentors and models for your child. Children with epilepsy who attend a special summer camp may experience an improvement in adaptive behaviors and social interactions. More information is available at www.efa.org.

12

EPILEPSY AND THE ELDERLY

Eleanor had a stroke at age seventy-six while recovering in the intensive care unit after a complicated heart operation. Her right arm and leg became weak, and she had difficulty finding the right words. After a month in a rehabilitation hospital, she regained all of her strength and went home with only a slight hesitancy of speech.

A few months later, while eating breakfast, Eleanor's right arm suddenly began jerking and she slumped over on the table unconscious. A minute or two later, she woke up and found pancakes in her lap. Her head hurt and she couldn't figure out what had happened. She got her neighbor to drive her to the emergency room. A computed axial tomography (CAT or CT) scan found evidence of her old stroke, but no new problem. Two weeks later, she had another spell. This time she bit her tongue and fell on the floor. After another visit to the hospital, a neurologic consultation, and an electroencephalogram (EEG), the doctors told her she had epilepsy.

152. Why do older people develop epilepsy?

Epilepsy is a disorder of neurons in the brain. Whenever these are damaged, seizures can result. While stroke is the most common cause of epilepsy in the elderly, other acquired insults to the brain such as brain tumors, dementia, head injury, and infections may also be responsible. People older than age seventy-five are at the greatest risk of developing epilepsy of any age group. More than 5% of nursing home residents have epilepsy.

When seizures occur in elderly patients, it is important to identify the underlying cause if possible. Most elderly people with seizures will need antiepileptic medication to control the seizures, as seizures are likely to recur in this age group.

153. What is the most common cause of epilepsy in the elderly?

As in Eleanor's case, new seizures in older people are most often caused by a cerebrovascular accident (stroke).

154. How can you determine the cause?

All patients with new-onset seizures, regardless of their age, must see a physician for a complete evaluation. This will consist of a history, physical and neurologic examinations, and usually an electroencephalograph (EEG) and brain scan, such as computed axial tomography (CAT or CT) or magnetic resonance imaging (MRI). However, even after a complete evaluation, the cause of new-onset epilepsy in the elderly remains unclear in 25 to 45% of cases.

Seizures may be more difficult to diagnose in elderly patients. For example, an epileptic seizure may be confused with a transient ischemic attack or fainting spell. After a seizure, older people may be confused for longer periods of time than younger patients. Neurologists experienced in the care of elderly people with epilepsy are aware of these diagnostic pitfalls.

155. So many older people get Alzheimer's disease. Can it cause epilepsy, too?

Yes. People with Alzheimer's disease have an increased risk of developing seizures.

156. What are other common causes of seizures in the elderly?

Brain tumors, head injury, and infections of the brain can cause seizures. Collections of blood that put pressure on the brain can also provoke seizures.

157. Is epilepsy treatment different in the elderly?

The principles of treatment are the same in the elderly as with younger patients. Treatment begins with identifying the cause of the seizures. For example, a seizure may be the first warning that a brain tumor is developing. Treatment of the tumor with surgery may eliminate the seizures. However, in many cases, there is no surgical cure for the cause of the seizures. Some brain tumors are inoperable, and there is no surgical treatment for the vast majority of strokes. In these situations, seizure control depends on antiepileptic medications.

Of course, when possible, an ounce of prevention is worth a pound of cure. For example, managing health problems like high blood pressure and high cholesterol may decrease the risk of stroke and the subsequent development of epilepsy.

158. Which are the best antiepileptic medications to use in older people?

The choice of antiepileptic medication for people with epilepsy is always complicated, especially in the elderly. The seizure type must first be identified, and your doctor will do this based on the clinical event, electroencephalogram (EEG), and brain scans such as computerized axial tomography (CAT or CT) and magnetic resonance imaging (MRI). Complex partial seizures are the most common seizure type in the elderly.

Another important consideration in elderly patients is the possibility for interactions with antiepileptic drugs and commonly used medications such as anticoagulants, calcium channel blockers, cimetidine, HMG-CoA reductase inhibitors (statins), quinidine, theophylline, and others. Potential drug-drug interactions are important to consider in any patient, but particularly in the elderly because they are likely to take multiple medications for various chronic medical problems. In a recent study, nearly 100% of elderly epilepsy patients were taking at least one other medication besides their epilepsy drug.

159. Are drug dosages the same in the elderly?

Typically, less medication is prescribed because drug metabolism is slower in older people. As people age, the liver and kidneys, responsible for most drug metabolism, do not work as well, which means that the dose of many medications must be reduced or toxic symptoms will result. Lower doses are also preferable because the elderly are more likely than younger patients to develop drowsiness or confusion from antiepileptic drugs. When treating older people with epilepsy, many neurologists try and avoid side effects by following the "low and slow" approach, beginning epilepsy drugs at a low dose and increasing the dose slowly over time as needed. The final maintenance dose is likely to be lower than for a younger patient.

160. How do you determine the right dose?

The right dose of antiepileptic medication is the least amount that controls the seizures and causes the fewest and mildest side effects. Accurate communication with your doctor, keeping your seizure calendar, regular doctor visits, and periodic measurement of serum drug levels are dependable ways to make sure you are taking the right dose. With the proper treatment, seizures are easily controlled in many elderly people with epilepsy.

161. How can I avoid drug interactions?

Once your dose is well regulated, it is important to inform your neurologist if one of your other doctors makes any changes in any of your other medications. For example, many elderly patients take phenytoin (Dilantin®) to control their seizures. Phenytoin is a very effective antiepileptic drug, but one that is liable to many drug-drug interactions. Phenytoin may lower the levels of atorvastatin (Lipitor®), a commonly used cholesterol-lowering drug. Conversely, cimetidine (Tagamet®) can raise the level of phenytoin, resulting in symptoms of toxicity. Three of the newer antiepileptic drugs, gabapentin (Neurontin®), levetiracetam (Keppra®), and pregabalin (Lyrica®), do not have clinically important drug-drug interactions and may be appropriate choices for elderly patients taking multiple medications. Keep your doctor up to date on your medications by bringing all your medication bottles to each office visit.

Whenever you are prescribed a new medicine, check with your physician and pharmacist to make sure there will be no undesirable drug-drug interactions. When you purchase a new medication from the pharmacy, the pharmacist will do a computer check to make sure the new prescription does not have an adverse reaction with any of your other medications. If you use several different pharmacies, make sure you give the pharmacist a list of all of your medications. Include over-the-counter and herbal medications as well (Chapter 6). Similarly, it is important to notify your doctor if you discontinue any of your medications, as this change may also have an effect on the drug levels of the remaining medications. You can write down any medication changes in the personal medical history section in the back of this book (Appendix A).

13

FIRST AID AND SAFETY TIPS

> I saw Carol for the first time in the emergency room. She was fumbling with the sheets on her stretcher and appeared confused. She didn't respond when I talked to her. I quickly interviewed her husband and began a neurological examination.
>
> Suddenly Carol's body stiffened and began to jerk. Her lips turned blue, and she bit her tongue. Blood trickled down her chin onto the pillow. I stood next to her and watched, making sure she didn't hurt herself. Her husband backed into the corner, horrified. The jerking stopped after what seemed like an hour, but was in fact only 90 seconds. After the convulsion, Carol took loud, deep, gurgling breaths. The nurse came in and helped me turn her on her side. I completed my examination, wrote admitting orders, and went to see my next patient.
>
> The following morning I got a call from the hospital administrator. Carol's husband was furious that I had allowed his wife to "have a seizure" and that "the doctor didn't do anything." The administrator demanded an explanation.

162. The patient had a seizure. Why didn't you do anything?

The most important thing to do during a seizure is to prevent patients from injuring themselves. When a patient has a convulsion, remove hard objects such as tables or chairs from their path. Protect their head by putting something soft under it, a pillow or jacket, even just your foot, so that the person's head does not bang on the floor or ground.

When you can, turn the person on his or her side to prevent saliva from blocking the airway. It is *not* advisable to stick something into the person's mouth. It is true that people can bite their tongue or cheeks during a convulsion. However, because this occurs early in the seizure, you are not likely to prevent it. Trying to force a spoon or stick between clenched teeth also risks breaking a tooth, which the patient may swallow or inhale. (Do not worry that the person will swallow their tongue. This does not occur. I have witnessed hundreds of convulsions, and we have not lost a tongue yet!) See Appendix J for a First Aid Checklist.

When people with epilepsy are confused during or after a seizure, prevent them from injury. Touch them as little as possible and do not restrain them. If you do, they may resist, and you will have a fight on your hands. Talk softly and be reassuring. Try not to be frightened.

Donna, a large woman on the epilepsy monitoring unit, started walking out of her room during a seizure, trailing her electroencephalograph wires behind her. This was potentially dangerous because she was hooked up with depth electrodes in her brain and running out of slack. As she approached me in the doorway, I gently turned her 180 degrees. She walked back into the room without missing a step.

Carol was on a stretcher with the guard rails up. She was in no danger of falling. My biggest concern was that she would strike her head, and I watched carefully to see that this did not happen. Her skin color and breathing improved promptly. During her seizure, I examined the jerking movements to see if there was any asymmetry that might point to a seizure focus.

I did not inject her with diazepam (Valium®) for two reasons. First, I would have had to leave her bedside to get it. Second, by the time I was ready, the seizure would have run its course, and the diazepam would have just made her sleepy.

I should have explained to her husband what had happened. At the time, I was preoccupied with getting Carol into the hospital and treating her to prevent another seizure. The next day she was fine and went home on antiepileptic medication. Before she left, I gave her and her husband first aid instructions and several pamphlets from the Epilepsy Foundation. I scheduled an appointment for them with the nurse at our comprehensive epilepsy center for additional epilepsy education. (I should probably have asked our hospital administrator to attend as well.)

163. When should I ask for an ambulance?

This is a judgment call. Knowing the patient makes the decision much easier. Jean has mild seizures characterized by slight confusion and humming. Her family has learned by experience that whenever her humming lasts longer than a few minutes, she will go on to have a tonic clonic convulsion. In her case, one convulsion leads to another and she develops status epilepticus. When Jean hums for more than a minute, they immediately take her to the emergency room.

One useful guideline for an observer is that the jerking and stiffening of a convulsion should not last more than two minutes. Any longer, and an ambulance should be called. If you can, time the seizure. A convulsion that lasts only a minute can seem a lot longer. Use a watch or clock to time it.

The drowsy phase after a seizure should not last longer than 15 minutes. By this time, patients should be alert enough to answer appropriately or say their names. Ask simple questions that require a specific answer. For example, "what day is it?," "where are you?," "tell me what is hurting you," and "how long have you had epilepsy?"

If you do not get a proper answer after 15 minutes, call an ambulance. (A reply of "OK" is not adequate evidence that the patient has recovered. After a seizure, Terry says "OK" to every question. If you ask, "are you all right?," he will say "OK." If you ask, "would you like to fly to the moon?," he will also say "OK.")

Check to see whether the patient has any injuries. Is there blood? Can the person walk without staggering? Because it is often difficult to know whether someone requires hospitalization, try to get some assistance with this decision. Call a family member or the patient's doctor. Check for a MedicAlert bracelet or necklace.

Most patients with epilepsy have single brief convulsions that do not require hospitalization. After the seizure, they may be confused for five or ten minutes. In addition, they may be tired, have sore muscles, and complain of a headache, but do not need immediate medical attention. Often they need to rest or go to sleep before resuming their normal activities.

Ask the person what he would like to do after a seizure. Does he want to go to the hospital? Does he want you to call his doctor? Does he need to find a ride? Tell him what happened. Be calm and supportive. A person with epilepsy may be embarrassed at having a seizure in public and may have soiled his clothes. Stay with him until he can take care of himself or someone else comes to help.

If it is a first seizure, call an ambulance. Anyone with a first seizure should go to the emergency room for a complete evaluation.

164. I live by myself and have convulsions about twice a month. I don't always have a warning. How can I make my home safer?

Years ago, when most homes were heated by open fires, many people with epilepsy sustained burns due to falls into the open hearth, resulting in many severe injuries. A few months ago, while working at a volunteer medical clinic in a Third World country, I saw such a patient. Although heating tends to be more modern now, burns from fireplaces, ovens, and hot water are still real problems in the United States and elsewhere.

Every home has two particularly dangerous areas, the kitchen and the bathroom. A number of minor modifications can decrease the likelihood of serious accidents:

KITCHEN

The short periods of confusion during and after a complex partial seizure predispose to injury. While cooking, you may place hands or arms on a gas or electric burner or spill hot food on yourself. In order to avoid this, use oven mitts and cook only on the rear burners.

An electric stove eliminates an open flame and the worry that you might leave the gas on. The safest option is to cook with a microwave. A microwave heats food behind a closed door and shuts off automatically. Microwave cookbooks are available.

To avoid dropping hot food during a seizure, keep a cart in the kitchen that you can wheel to the table.

Tap water can become hot enough to scald. Ask your plumber to install a heat control device in the kitchen faucet to prevent the water from becoming dangerously hot.

Consider carpeting the kitchen floor. Although not as easy to clean, it is much more comfortable to land on.

Whenever possible, use plastic containers rather than glass.

BATHROOM

One of my patients let the hot water run in the tub during a seizure and severely burned both feet. This type of injury can be prevented by installing a temperature control device in the tub and shower heads.

There are many hard surfaces in the bathroom—the sink, the tub, the toilet—that you can't do much about, but you can carpet the floor. Carpet is softer and less slippery than tile.

Do not put a lock on the bathroom door. If you have one, don't use it. It will be difficult for someone to help you after a seizure if they cannot get in.

Learn to take a bath with only a few inches of water in the tub. Use a hand-held shower head and shower while sitting. If you have frequent seizures, bathe with supervision.

Stairs can be dangerous. If possible, choose a ranch house or one-floor apartment rather than a townhouse. If you have stairs, try to arrange your routine to limit how often you must go from floor to floor.

Use more carpet! Avoid shiny hardwood floors.

If you have a fireplace, keep a protective screen in front of it.

Irons can get very hot. Buy one that shuts off automatically. Avoid curling irons. They give a nasty burn.

Another household hazard is cigarettes. To decrease the risk of fire, do not smoke in the house. Better yet, do not smoke! Install smoke alarms in each room.

See Appendix I for a Home Safety Checklist.

Some people have "seizure-alert" or "seizure-response" dogs that may alert them when they are going to have a seizure or stay close to them after a seizure. These service dogs require a great deal of training and commitment from their owners (Appendix H).

165. My seizures usually occur early in the morning when I have stayed up late. What can I do?

Some patients know when they are likely to have seizures. Certain circumstances, such as sleep deprivation, missed anti-epileptic medication, or time of the month, may herald the onset of a convulsion. An increase in myoclonic jerks may suggest that a generalized tonic clonic seizure will soon follow.

On days when they are at high risk for seizures because of sleep deprivation, I ask my patients to stay in bed a little longer. If they do have a convulsion, it will happen in a soft bed, not while running across the street to catch a bus. If they have missed their antiepileptic medication, they need to make it up. If it is a high-risk time of the month, they should avoid potentially dangerous activities such as bicycle riding or boating.

A little prevention can eliminate the need for a lot of first aid.

An animated review of epilepsy first aid is available at www.epilepsy.com.

14

CLINICAL RESEARCH:
Should I Participate
in a Drug Trial?

J im is a thirty-five-year-old man I have treated for five years. He has
partial complex seizures about 12 times a month. First he notices an
aura of a heavy feeling in his tongue, and then he will stare, chew, cough,
and become confused. Sometimes he falls. He has broken a rib and
fractured both great toes due to seizures.

Despite trying five antiepileptic medications, his seizures continued. We observed him in the epilepsy monitoring unit and discovered
that the seizures began in at least three separate regions of his brain.
Consequently, he was not a candidate for a surgical resection. His
mother, who still looks after him, asked me whether there was anything
else we could try.

Three years ago, Jim enrolled in a clinical trial in order to try an
investigational antiepileptic drug. His seizure frequency has slightly
reduced; down to eight a month. He and his mother also told me that
the seizures are briefer and less severe. The only side effect he has from
the protocol medication is a tremor.

166. What is a drug trial?

Before a new epilepsy medication can be released on the
market, the manufacturer must demonstrate to the Food and
Drug Administration (FDA) that the medication is safe and
effective. In order to do this, new medications are first tested in
animals, then in healthy human volunteers, then in people with

epilepsy. All human testing must be approved by the FDA. Each study design must also be approved by an institutional review board (IRB) composed of health care professionals and lay persons to ensure that the study meets ethical standards. Patients must be fully informed of all the risks and benefits and great care is taken to protect their safety.

It may be some comfort to patients with difficult to control epilepsy to learn that many people are involved in the search for new and better treatments for epilepsy. Pharmaceutical companies spend billions of dollars in laboratories and clinics in the United States and many other countries to achieve this goal. Clinical trials are very painstaking work and the only road to scientifically proven treatments for epilepsy. For example, ten years ago, I was a principal investigator for an epilepsy drug that had shown much promise in early trials. However, in our more rigorous study, patients failed to show any benefit from the drug, and the company abandoned its development. Another drug I tested in a clinical trial later became the most successful epilepsy drug on the market. Over the years, I have had the opportunity both to participate in clinical research and interview many researchers at neurology conferences. I have been very impressed by their hard work, dedication, and expertise. The work of clinical investigators (and patient volunteers!) has resulted in FDA approval of ten new antiepileptic drugs and the vagus nerve stimulator in the last fifteen years. Many other new drugs are currently in development for the control of epileptic seizures (Appendix B) as well as an implanted electrical stimulator (Question #180).

167. Why doesn't my doctor prescribe one of the new drugs for me?

An investigational drug can only be given to a patient during a clinical trial. It cannot be prescribed until it receives Food and Drug Administration (FDA) approval.

An investigational drug study requires a huge commitment of time and energy from each patient as well as the physician and nurses conducting the study. Patients must record each seizure carefully and take each dose of medication exactly as directed. To check on compliance, at each visit a nurse will count all the pills left in the medication bottles. Trips to the doctor are frequent and can be lengthy (often two hours or more).

After the FDA has approved the study, the principal investigator (PI) at each site must attend a conference at which the study goals and limitations are discussed. Then the physician must justify the project to the institutional review board (IRB), keep careful records (typically in triplicate), repeatedly examine patients in great detail, and review hundreds of pages of laboratory data. The clinical site must pass inspection by the pharmaceutical company and prepare for possible examination by the FDA.

Because of the amount of organization, facilities, and time required for a drug study, this type of epilepsy research is usually performed at medical schools or comprehensive epilepsy centers (Appendix D).

168. What is a drug protocol?

A protocol is a specific plan that spells out exactly how the research will be performed. Each drug study has its own protocol, which must be followed exactly for the results to have scientific value. For example, the protocol dictates the medication dose patients receive, how often they must come for a check-up, the number of weeks of the study, and which type of testing is necessary, such as electroencephalograms (EEGs), electrocardiograms (EKGs), blood tests, and urine samples.

Most epilepsy clinical trials are performed at several locations, or sites. By following the protocol, the doctors at each site perform the study exactly the same way. In this manner, all the information collected can be pooled for analysis when the trial is completed.

169. When should I consider a drug study?

For most patients, a drug study should be considered when conventional therapy has failed, either because seizures are not controlled or side effects are intolerable. Jim had already tried most of the available antiepileptic medications, and he was not a surgical candidate. A clinical trial held the promise of a new drug that might be helpful, but would not be available by prescription for years. Additionally, Jim and his mother would get the reassurance of frequent doctor visits and blood monitoring. Another benefit of enrolling in a drug study is the satisfaction of knowing that the results of this clinical research will help other people with epilepsy. There is no guarantee that you will personally benefit when you participate in a clinical trial.

170. How do I know it is safe?

Part of the purpose of a drug study is to determine whether the new antiepileptic medication causes side effects in patients. Consequently, there is no guarantee that the drug is safe. However, patient safety is "Job #1" in any clinical trial. The patient's safety is more important than any study result. In addition, we learn from side effects. If a new antiepileptic drug controls seizures, but has severe side effects, it won't receive Food and Drug Administration (FDA) approval.

In order to protect patients, study protocols typically require frequent doctor visits during which the patient receives a physical and neurological examination as well as blood and urine tests. Patients are encouraged to keep in close contact by phone. Clinical trial investigators always provide a contact number that can be used 24 hours/day. In this manner, if there is a dangerous side effect, it will be found early. In my experience, serious problems are rare.

There are definite risks to participating in a drug study including possible allergic and other adverse reactions to the new antiepileptic drug. However, the risk for patients with intractable epilepsy of *not* participating is likely to be continued uncontrolled seizures.

171. How much does it cost to participate in a study?

In most instances, the cost of the investigational medication, clinic visits, and laboratory testing is borne by the pharmaceutical sponsor. In other words, the study is free. For people with epilepsy who don't have medical insurance, a clinical trial provides an opportunity for very thorough medical care with little, if any, out-of-pocket cost. Patients may receive a small amount of compensation to cover travel or other study-related costs.

172. Can I stop in the middle of the study?

Patients can stop participating in a study at any time and for any reason. Patients usually withdraw from studies only if they have a severe adverse reaction to the investigational drug or if it fails to help them. (You should never begin a study if you are not convinced it is the right thing to do.)

173. What kind of results should I expect from a drug study?

Jim's story is fairly typical. He did not experience a dramatic improvement in his seizures, but they are now occurring less often and are less severe. He is somewhat better. Some patients do not benefit at all from a new drug, and a few get worse, but every study is begun with the hope that the new drug represents an improvement over all the other available treatment options.

174. How do I know if there is a protocol drug that might help me?

If your seizures remain uncontrolled and your doctor has exhausted new treatment options, you should ask your doctor for a referral to a comprehensive epilepsy center or other research facility (Appendix D). There you will be evaluated to determine whether you fit the inclusion and exclusion criteria of the particular study. For example, in one of our studies, in order to be included a patient must be between fifteen and seventy years old and have partial complex seizures at least three times a month. Patients are excluded if they are pregnant, have severe medical or psychiatric disease, abuse drugs or alcohol, or are noncompliant.

If you qualify for the study, the details will be explained to you, as well as potential risks, benefits, and costs. Then you can decide whether you want to participate.

175. What is informed consent?

Informed consent is an ethical concept that presumes an individual to be the best person to make a decision regarding his or her own care. Before you enroll in a study, the possible risks to your health, potential benefits from the drug, and alternatives to the study must be discussed with you. The Food and Drug Administration (FDA) requires that you sign an informed consent form in order to begin a drug trial to demonstrate that you understand what the study is about, why you should be in it, what will happen during the study, and that you freely agree to participate.

176. What is an open-label trial?

In many clinical trials, the name and amount of experimental drug are known to the investigator and the patient. This is an open-label trial.

A study in which the investigator or patient does not know whether an investigational drug or placebo is being used is a "blinded" trial. When both the doctor and the patient are not allowed to know whether the patient is receiving the active drug or placebo, the trial is called "double-blind."

177. What is a "placebo effect"?

In certain drug study protocols, some patients receive active drug while others receive an inactive substance, or placebo. The placebo is designed to look like the study drug.

For reasons that remain mysterious, under the proper circumstances, some patients improve with anything new, usually temporarily. Sarah is a twenty-year-old patient of mine with a behavior disorder and frequent seizures (as often as 26 times a month). After trials of seven different epilepsy drugs failed to control her seizures, she reluctantly entered a drug trial. The first phase of the study required her to begin with a placebo, or sugar pill. When she returned for follow-up a month later, Sarah exclaimed she had not had one seizure! According to her mother, even her behavior was much improved. She had responded to the power of suggestion, not to a miracle drug.

178. What is a "double-blind" trial?

In a "single blind" study, the doctor knows whether the patient is taking the investigational drug or the placebo, but the patient does not. In a "double-blind" study, neither the doctor nor the patient knows. Records are kept in code. At the end of the trial, the "blind is broken" and the results are analyzed. The seizure frequency of the two groups is compared to see whether the new drug helped patients more than the placebo. The purpose of "blinding" the study is to prevent the possibility of bias from affecting the results.

179. Will my doctor be upset if I don't participate?

You should not feel any pressure to enter a drug study. If you are an appropriate candidate, it is natural for your doctor to encourage you.

I have been frustrated by one of my patients who continues to have many seizures a month. She refuses to try an investigational antiepileptic medication because of the "risks." She does not seem to understand that there are also real risks to her continued seizures. In addition to the adverse effects on her quality of life, she may be injured or even die as a result of her continued seizures. I think she would do much better with a protocol antiepileptic medication. Maybe someday she will change her mind and we will find out.

180. Are there any other options for Jim since the new drug doesn't work?

Many new investigational epilepsy drugs are currently under investigation (Appendix B). Some of these new drugs are structurally similar to antiepileptic drugs already on the market and may result in improved versions with better efficacy or less side effects. Others are completely new formulations. Jim is comfortable now with his improvement and not ready to try something new. However, if he would like to, he can choose to enroll in a different drug trial. If he starts a new trial, he will have to stop the investigational antiepileptic drug he is taking, as it is too complicated for patients to be in more than one clinical trial at the same time.

In addition to new antiepileptic drugs, there are several types of brain stimulation under investigation for epilepsy treatment. Transcranial magnetic stimulation is a novel approach for the treatment of epilepsy. It uses a magnetic pulse generated by a metal coil held near the head. Another type of brain stimulation with direct electrical current is also being evaluated. Very little electrical current is used. Both of these techniques stimulate the brain from outside the skull.

Experiments with deep brain stimulation are also ongoing using a battery-powered stimulator that is implanted inside the brain. This type of brain research is limited to people whose seizures cannot be controlled any other way (intractable epilepsy). One device under investigation, the NeuroPace RNS System, uses the principle of responsive stimulation; first it detects a seizure and then it sends an electrical stimulation to stop it. (You won't feel the electrical stimulation.) The stimulator is programmed with a laptop computer. A pivotal clinical trial of the NeuroPace RNS Neurostimulator for patients with intractable and disabling partial seizures is currently underway at more than 20 epilepsy centers. More information is available at www.seizurestudy.com or (866) 903-2437.

Other options for patients with intractable epilepsy include the ketogenic and modified Atkins diets (Question #147), epilepsy surgery (Chapter 7), and the vagus nerve stimulator (Question #73). The vagus nerve stimulator received FDA approval in 1997.

More information regarding ongoing trials for new epilepsy treatments can be found at www.clinicaltrials.gov and www.centerwatch.com.

15

WHO ELSE CAN HELP?

> S andy had seizures since infancy. She described a "feeling from
> behind" like a "wave." Then she would become confused. On rare
> occasions, she had a grand mal convulsion. Over the years, she tried
> nine antiepileptic medications to control her seizures, and she still had
> about three seizures a month. Her electroencephalographs (EEGs) and
> magnetic resonance imaging (MRI) pointed to a seizure focus in her
> right temporal lobe.
>   When I recommended epilepsy surgery, she became frightened and
> didn't return to see me for nearly a year. It was only because of the
> repeated urging of her friend who had already had seizure surgery that
> she came back. Last year, she consented to a right temporal lobectomy.
> Today, she is seizure-free.

181. Should I go to a support group?

Not everyone has a knowledgeable, supportive friend like
Sandy. If your seizures are causing problems at home, at work,
or with transportation, you may want to attend a support group
to benefit from the experience of other people with epilepsy.
Without her friend's encouragement, Sandy might never have
returned for another look at surgery.

A support group can be very helpful. Others in your
community with epilepsy are likely to know which pharmacy has
the lowest medication prices, have opinions on the best epilepsy
doctors, and recommend the most responsive social agencies.

Many people also feel better when they meet others who
understand the experience of seizures and deal with similar

issues. Groups often help to increase social support and reduce feelings of isolation. In some cases, patients discover that their epilepsy is much milder than others in the support group.

If your seizures are well controlled and epilepsy does not interfere with your life, you do not need a support group. You may wish to go in order to help others become as well adjusted as you are.

182. I would be more comfortable talking to people with epilepsy outside my community. What can I do?

Be on the lookout for conferences for people with epilepsy sponsored by a variety of organizations such as the Epilepsy Foundation and FACES (Finding A Cure for Epilepsy and Seizures). In addition, chat forums are available on the internet, such as the ones at www.epilepsy.com and www.epilepsyfoundation.org, which allow you to communicate with others who have epilepsy outside of your community.

183. What about a counselor?

Many patients benefit from discussing their problems with a clinical psychologist or other trained counselor. According to one epilepsy specialist, nearly all patients with epilepsy and their families require counseling sometime along the way. Modern life is stressful, and uncontrolled seizures compound daily problems. Not being able to drive or work puts pressure on people with epilepsy and their families. A psychologist, social worker, or other health care professional may help people with epilepsy deal more effectively with these challenges. Counselors may also be available at school or church.

Comorbid psychiatric conditions such as anxiety and depression frequently occur in people with epilepsy, especially those with uncontrolled seizures. These psychiatric problems may need to be treated by a psychiatrist, psychologist, or other health care professional. If you feel anxious, depressed, or hopeless, tell your doctor, who will explore ways to treat these conditions or refer you to someone who can.

184. What about a social worker?

Comprehensive epilepsy centers and hospitals employ social workers who can assist you with transportation, funding, and counseling. A social worker is an excellent community resource. For example, some patients may qualify for disability or Medicaid, but need help in the application process. Special transportation may be available that you may not know about. If you cannot find a social worker in your area, try the Epilepsy Information Service hotline for more information (800-642-0500).

185. My doctor is always so busy, and I have so many questions! Whom do I ask?

Not all of your questions need to be answered by your doctor. In my office, trained nurses and medical office assistants answer most patient questions over the telephone. We also distribute educational pamphlets that discuss common problems such as epilepsy first aid, neurological testing, and driving. I try to answer difficult or complex questions during office visits. Many doctors provide educational information on their websites, and some doctors will respond to questions by email.

If you would like your doctor to answer your questions, write them down and bring the list to your next office visit. Explain to your doctor at the beginning of your visit that you have some very important questions, and your doctor will make time to answer them. If possible, bring someone along with you to help remember the answers (Chapter 3).

For more general questions, find the address of your local Epilepsy Foundation affiliate (Appendix C) and ask about an epilepsy education class. See if there is a comprehensive epilepsy center nearby (Appendix D). Your pharmacist will be happy to provide printed information about your epilepsy medication. Antiepileptic drug information is also provided on the manufacturers' websites (Appendix B).

Check the bibliography for books that interest you. Try the public library. Excellent books, pamphlets, and videos are available from the Epilepsy Foundation catalog. The Epilepsy Foundation also maintains an outstanding library.

Support groups and epilepsy societies exist all over the world (Appendix G). There are even internet websites devoted to epilepsy and the human brain (Appendix H). Appendix K lists other resources that may be helpful as well.

186. What about vocational rehabilitation (VR)?

If you are unemployed, ask your doctor for a referral to vocational rehabilitation. They will assess your skills and may arrange job training. Vocational rehabilitation can determine whether it is practical for you to work and help you find an appropriate job.

187. I have trouble taking care of myself, doing chores, and looking after the children, particularly since I can't drive anywhere, but I can't afford any help. What can I do?

One of my patients with severe memory problems obtained considerable home assistance for her new baby from the members of her church. Many religious congregations feel that it is their responsibility to care for the needy. Talk to your pastor, rabbi, or other religious leader about your situation. At the very least, you may find some spiritual support. In addition, some counties have programs to assist with different needs. You may want to contact your county department of disability services.

188. What about legal help? I'm concerned that I may lose my job because of epilepsy.

The Americans with Disabilities Act provides job protection for people with epilepsy in certain circumstances. Some attorneys provide free (pro bono) assistance as a public service or you may qualify for legal aid. Contact your Epilepsy Foundation affiliate for information on local legal resources (Appendix C).

189. I've been seeing my family doctor for five years. He has tried me on several antiepileptic medications, but I keep having seizures. Isn't there anything else I can do?

It may be time for a referral to a neurologist who specializes in epilepsy management (epileptologist) or to a comprehensive epilepsy center (Appendix D). There have been significant advances in the last five years in the management of epilepsy, and the newest treatments are only available at epilepsy centers. Tell your doctor how much you appreciate working with him and ask whether you might benefit from seeing an epilepsy specialist as well. If your seizures are not controlled, chances are your doctor is as frustrated as you and will embrace this suggestion. Even if you see an epilepsy specialist, try and keep a good relationship with your family doctor, who knows you well and is closer to home.

16

NONEPILEPTIC
SEIZURES

When I met Katherine at the hospital, she was twenty years old, four months pregnant, and homeless. She had a history of depression, physical and sexual abuse, and three suicide attempts. She was separated from her husband and lived in a shelter for pregnant women. Several months earlier, Kathy was injured in a fight with her boyfriend. Her father was going to testify against the boyfriend but died of a heart attack while waiting for the trial. Her mother blamed Kathy for her father's death, became depressed, and committed suicide. Then Kathy was hospitalized for depression. The workers at the shelter said she had behavior problems and was difficult to manage.

Kathy's seizures began at the age of 5, but she received no treatment until age 18. Eventually, one doctor prescribed carbamazepine (Tegretol®), which made her wobbly and sleepy, so she stopped it. Then she began divalproex sodium (Depakote®), which she tolerated better, but she continued to have breakthrough seizures. When Kathy discovered she was pregnant, at ten weeks, she discontinued the anti-epileptic medication. Her seizure frequency increased, resulting in two emergency room visits and now this hospital admission to the epilepsy monitoring unit. Kathy's neurological exam and magnetic resonance imaging (MRI) were normal.

Over several days, we recorded five of her seizures on the closed circuit television and electroencephalograph (CCTV/EEG) monitoring equipment. She appeared to lose consciousness during each spell. In one of them, she had dramatic jerking, pelvic thrusting, grimacing, and crying. Not one of the EEGs showed any epileptic activity. I explained to her that she had nonepileptic seizures, or pseudoseizures. Kathy had trouble accepting that her spells resulted from the significant social stresses in her life and not from epilepsy.

190. What is a pseudoseizure?

Some people experience spells that resemble epileptic seizures. They may stare and be unresponsive, or even jerk and salivate. In epileptic seizures, there is always a distinctive electrical discharge from neurons in the brain, which can usually be seen on the electroencephalogram (EEG). In pseudoseizures, the brain waves reveal no epileptic activity.

191. How can you tell if a patient is having a pseudoseizure or an epileptic seizure?

Sometimes an experienced neurologist can tell by watching the patient closely. Certain types of behaviors are rare in true epileptic seizures, but far more common in nonepileptic ones. A more reliable method is to monitor the person with video and electroencephalography (EEG) and record the spells. Then the video can be studied in detail as well as the EEG. Using this method, we are able to accurately diagnose 90% of patients. At a busy comprehensive epilepsy center, 20 to 30% of patients who come for monitoring may have nonepileptic seizures. Before coming in for this specialized monitoring, many patients with nonepileptic seizures have been misdiagnosed with epilepsy for five to ten years!

Another method that may also help distinguish epileptic from nonepileptic seizures is the measurement of prolactin, a hormone that is released from the brain in greater quantities after a convulsion or partial complex seizure. A blood test for prolactin may be taken a few minutes after a seizure and again twenty-four hours later for comparison. If the prolactin level is significantly higher after the seizure, it suggests that the seizure may be epileptic.

192. Why would someone fake a seizure?

In most cases, the patient is unaware that the seizure is not epileptic. To the patient, the seizure is real. Most people with nonepileptic seizures experience significant psychosocial stress in their lives and have limited coping skills and poor family support. Katherine's case history is a good example of a person who is at risk for developing nonepileptic seizures. Because psychological problems are often the underlying problem, pseudoseizures are sometimes called psychogenic seizures.

193. What would make you suspect a patient has pseudoseizures?

Sometimes the clinical history is suggestive with an unusual time course, bizarre seizure types, or failure to respond to antiepileptic medications, especially when seen in a patient who has obvious psychological problems. It was peculiar, for example, that Kathy had seizures throughout most of her life, but no antiepileptic medications were prescribed until she was eighteen years old. She was also in a high-risk group for pseudoseizures; that is, women of childbearing age with a history of physical and sexual abuse.

194. I have never heard of pseudoseizures. How common a problem is it?

In my specialized epilepsy practice, I saw one hundred and sixty cases over five years, so it is not rare. But the vast majority of people with seizures have epilepsy, not pseudoseizures.

195. Can pseudoseizures occur in children or the elderly?

Yes. They can occur at most any age. I have seen patients with pseudoseizures in their eighties.

196. Are there other causes of pseudoseizures besides psychiatric disease?

Yes. Sometimes people have other medical problems that mimic epileptic seizures. They can be challenging to diagnose. For example, I took care of one patient with diabetes who would occasionally feel sleepy, slump over, and become stiff. When we monitored her on the epilepsy unit, her blood sugars were normal and there was no epileptic activity on the electroencephalograph (EEG). Initially, the problem appeared psychological. However, after studying her more closely, we discovered that she had a severe diabetic autonomic neuropathy. Unexpected drops in blood pressure lowered the flow of oxygen to her brain, causing her to pass out. In this case, treatment was medical, not psychological.

197. Do epilepsy medications help treat pseudoseizures?

No. Antiepileptic medications such as carbamazepine (Tegretol®), divalproex sodium (Depakote®), phenytoin (Dilantin®), phenobarbital, or any of the newer antiepileptic drugs do not control pseudoseizures. One great value of making the correct diagnosis of pseudoseizures is that patients can be protected from the cost and health risks of taking antiepileptic medications that they do not need. Kathy suffered side effects from carbamazepine and her baby risked birth defects from valproic acid. Both medications were intended to treat epilepsy, a disorder she did not have!

198. How do you treat pseudoseizures?

The first part of treatment is making an accurate diagnosis. This can only be done reliably by a specialist in epilepsy with the use of electroencephalography (EEG) and typically takes place at an epilepsy center. Once the diagnosis is made, it must be carefully explained to the patient and family. Patients are often reluctant to accept that they have a psychiatric disease instead of a medical disorder like epilepsy. Epilepsy medication is slowly withdrawn. The patients must enter into therapy with a psychiatrist or psychologist. If the patients have significant psychiatric illness, such as depression or anxiety, the psychiatrist may prescribe specific medication.

Group therapy sessions for patients with pseudoseizures may be helpful. These provide an opportunity for the discussion of the diagnosis, evaluation of psychosocial stressors, and keeping track of the "seizures." Many patients find support in knowing there are others with the same unusual problem.

199. Can a patient have both epileptic and nonepileptic seizures?

Yes, although this does not occur often. One study suggested that only one in ten patients with pseudoseizures also had epilepsy. As you may imagine, these patients are difficult to treat. They require both antiepileptic medications and psychotherapy.

Afterword

I hope you enjoyed reading this book. Now that you know the answers to these 199 questions, you can manage your epilepsy with greater understanding and success.

Advances in epilepsy treatment continue at a rapid pace.

Because of continued progress in the treatment of epilepsy, another updated edition of *Epilepsy: 199 Answers* is inevitable if the information is to stay current. If you have questions that you think should be included in future editions, please visit my website at:

www.drwilner.org

If this book has helped you to control your seizures, please share your story with me.

In the meantime, work closely with your doctor and health care team, take advantage of the many helpful resources listed in this book, and good luck in controlling your seizures!

Andrew N. Wilner, MD, FACP, FAAN

My Health Record

Personal Medical History

Have you ever had any of the following problems? (If you do not know, check with family members and try to complete this list before you see your neurologist.)

- Problems at birth? Premature? Low birth weight? Needed an incubator?
- Problems with development? How old were you when you learned to walk and talk?
- How much school did you complete?
- Did you require special classes?
- Encephalitis (infection in the brain)?
- Meningitis (infection in the coverings of the brain)?
- Head injury with loss of consciousness?
- Febrile seizures (seizures with fever as an infant or young child)?
- Family member with epilepsy?
- Allergies to medications or injections?
- Medical illness requiring hospitalization?
- Psychiatric illness (depression, hallucinations)?
- Problem with drugs or alcohol?
- Surgery?

- Can you describe your seizure? Ask a friend or family member to help you:
    - Do you have a warning?
    - Do you have a convulsion?
    - Do you stare?
    - Do you lose control of your urine?
    - Do you bite your tongue?
    - Are you tired after a seizure?
    - Do you have a headache afterwards?
    - How often do they occur?
    - Are they more frequent around the time of your period?
    - Do seizures happen only at night?
    - Does anything seem to trigger your seizures?

Write down the medications you take for epilepsy, the dose in milligrams, and when you take them:

Time of Day	Medication #1	Medication #2	Medication #3	Medication #4
Morning				
Noon				
Supper				
Bedtime				

- Do these medications completely control your seizures? Yes/No
- Do these medications give you any troublesome side effects? Yes/No
- If you have side effects, what are they?

Do you take any other medications for other health problems? List them here:

1.
2.
3.

Write down any herbal or alternative medicine therapies you are taking:

1.
2.
3.

Write down any antiepileptic medications you have tried for epilepsy in the past that did not work:

1.
2.
3.

If you have had any of the following tests, write down the results if you know them:

Magnetic resonance imaging (MRI):

_____

Computed axial tomography (CAT or CT) scan:

_____

Electroencephalograph (EEG):

_____

Important Telephone Numbers

1. Medical doctor:
2. Neurologist:
3. Pharmacist:
4. Supervisor at work:
5. Closest family member:
6. Friend who drives:
7. Person to call in emergency:

My Seizure Calendar

1. Photocopy the calendar on the next page.
2. Write in the name of the month and the dates.
3. Mark the letter "C" if you have a convulsion.
4. Mark the letter "S" if you have a staring spell.
5. Put the letter "M" if you missed medication.
6. Put the letter "D" if you are dizzy, have double vision, or other side effects.
7. Add other information if you think it is important, such as the days of your menstrual period, headaches, other illnesses, or stressful events in your life.
8. Bring this calendar with you every time you see your doctor.

Month

Monday	Tuesday	Wednesday	Thursday	Friday	Saturday	Sunday

B

Medications for the Treatment of Epilepsy and Pharmaceutical and Device Contact Information

Medications for the Treatment of Epilepsy

BRAND NAME	GENERIC
Carbatrol	carbamazepine extended release
Celontin	methsuximide
Cerebyx	fosphenytoin
Dilantin	phenytoin
Depakene	valproic acid
Depakote	divalproex sodium
Depakote ER	divalproex sodium extended release
Diamox	acetazolamide
Felbatol	felbamate
Gabitril	tiagabine
Keppra	levetiracetam
Klonopin	clonazepam
Lamictal	lamotrigine

Lyrica   pregabalin
Mebaral   mephobarbital
Mysoline   primidone
Neurontin   gabapentin
Phenobarbital   phenobarbital
Tegretol   carbamazepine
Tegretol XR   carbamazepine extended release
Topamax   topiramate
Tranzene   clorazepate
Trileptal   oxcarbazepine
Zarontin   ethosuximide
Zonegran   zonisamide

Investigational Antiepileptic Medications*

BRAND NAME	GENERIC
Pending	brivaracetam (UCB 34714)
Pending	carisbamate (RWJ-333369)
Frisium	clobazam
Pending	DP-VPA
Pending	eslicarbazepine acetate (BIA 2-093)
Pending	fluorofelbamate
Pending	ganaxolone
Pending	ICA-105665
Pending	isovaleramide
Pending	lacosamide
Keppra XR	levetiracetam extended release
Pending	muscimol

*These are research drugs for the treatment of epilepsy in various phases of development. As of August 2007, they have not been approved by the Food and Drug Administration (FDA).

Pending	retigabine
Inovelon	rufinamide
Pending	safinamide
Pending	selectracetam (UCB 44212)
Rapamycin	sirolimus
Pending	stiripentol
Pending	talampanel
Pending	valrocemide
Sabril	vigabatrin

Pharmaceutical and Device Information Resources

These numbers and web sites may help your doctor obtain information about pharmaceutical company–sponsored indigent programs or answer specific inquiries about medications.

- Abbott Laboratories (Depacon, Depakote, Depakote ER), www.abbott.com, (800) 255-5162
- Cephalon Professional Services (Gabitril), www.cephalon.com, (800) 896-5855
- Cyberonics, Inc. (Vagus Nerve Stimulator), www.cyberonics.com, (800) 332-1375
- Eisai (Zonegran), www.eisai.com, (201) 692-1100
- GlaxoSmithKline (Lamictal), www.gsk.com, (888) 825 5249
- MedPointe (Felbatol), www.medpointepharma.com, (732) 564-2200
- Novartis (Tegretol, Tegretol XR, Trileptal), www.novartis.com, (888) 644-8585
- Ortho-McNeil Pharmaceuticals (Topamax), www.ortho-mcneil.com, (800) 682-6532
- Ovation (Mebaral), www.ovationpharma.com, (866) 209-7604

- Pfizer (Celontin, Dilantin, Lyrica, Neurontin, Zarontin), www.pfizer.com, (800) 438-1985
- Roche Laboratories (Klonopin), www.roche.com, (800) 526-6367
- Shire US, Inc. (Carbatrol), www.shire.com, (800) 536-7878
- UCB Pharma (Keppra), www.ucbepilepsy.com, (800) 477-7877

Resource Guide

National Epilepsy Associations

Epilepsy Foundation
8301 Professional Place, East
Landover, MD 20785
Information Service
(800) 332-1000, (301) 459-3700
www.epilepsyfoundation.org

Epilepsy Foundation National Epilepsy Library Database
(800) 332-4050
FAX: (301) 577-4941
nel@efa.org

American Epilepsy Society
642 North Main Street
West Hartford, CT 06117-2507
(860) 586-7505
FAX: (860) 586-7550
info@aesnet.org
www.aesnet.org

State Epilepsy Associations

· ALABAMA

Epilepsy Foundation of North and Central Alabama
1900 Crestwood Boulevard,
Suite 96
Birmingham, AL 35210-2056
(205) 951-4151, (800) 950-6662
FAX: (205) 951-4152
epilepsy@aol.com

Epilepsy Foundation of South Alabama
951 Government Street,
Suite 201
Mobile, AL 36604-2425
(251) 432-0970, (800) 626-1582
FAX: (251) 432-0975
info@epilepsysouthalabama.org

· ARIZONA

Epilepsy Foundation of Arizona
P.O. Box 25084
Phoenix, AZ 85002-5084
(602) 406-3581, (888) 768-2690
FAX: (602) 406-6147
mmaclei@chw.edu

· CALIFORNIA

**Epilepsy Foundation of
Northern California**
5700 Stoneridge Mall Road, Suite 295
Pleasanton, CA 94588-2852
(925) 224-7760, (800) 632-3532
FAX: (925) 224-7770
efnca@epilepsynorcal.org

**Epilepsy Foundation of
San Diego County**
2055 El Cajon Boulevard
San Diego, CA 92104-1091
(619) 296-0161
FAX: (619) 296-0802
info@epilepsysandiego.org

**Epilepsy Foundation of Greater
Los Angeles**
577 West Century Boulevard,
Suite 820
Los Angeles, CA 90045-9007
(310) 670-2870, (800) 564-0445
FAX: (310) 670-6124
pietsch@epilepsy-socalif.org

· COLORADO

Epilepsy Foundation of Colorado
234 Columbine Street, Suite 333
Denver, CO 80206-4711
(303) 377-9774, (888) 378-9779
FAX: (303) 377-0081
gail@epilepsycolorado.org

· CONNECTICUT

**Epilepsy Foundation of
Connecticut**
386 Main Street
Middletown, CT 06457-3360
(860) 346-1924, (800) 899-3745
FAX: (860) 346-1928
1wallace.efct@sbcglobal.net

· DELAWARE

Epilepsy Foundation of Delaware
New Castle Corporate Commons
Tower Office Park
240 North James St, Suite 208
Newport, DE 19804-3171
(302) 999-9313, (800) 422-3653
FAX: (302) 999-9763
efd@efde.org

· FLORIDA

Epilepsy Foundation of Florida
7300 N Kendall Drive, Suite 700
Miami, FL 33156-7840
(305) 670-4949
FAX: (305) 670-0904
kegozi@efosf.org

· GEORGIA

Epilepsy Foundation of Georgia
6065 Roswell Road, #515
Atlanta, GA 30328-4015
(404) 527-7155, (800) 527-7105
FAX: (404) 564-3034
charlottethompson@mindspring.com

· HAWAII

Epilepsy Foundation of Hawaii
501 Sumner Street, P.H. 4
Honolulu, HI 96817
(808) 528-3058
FAX: (808) 528-3103
director-efh@hawaiiepilepsy.com

· IDAHO

Epilepsy Foundation of Idaho
310 West Idaho Street
Boise, ID 83702-6039
(208) 344-4340, (800) 237-6676
FAX: (208) 343-0093
efid@epilepsyidaho.org

· ILLINOIS

**Epilepsy Foundation of
North/Central Illinois, Iowa,
and Nebraska**
321 West State Street, Suite 208
Rockford, IL 61101-1119
(815) 964-2689, (800) 221-2689
FAX: (815) 964-2731
efncil@efncil.org

**Epilepsy Foundation of
Greater Chicago**
17 N State Street, Suite 1300
Chicago, IL 60602-3297
(312) 939-8622, (800) 273-6027
FAX: (312) 939-0391
info@epilepsychicago.org

**Epilepsy Foundation of Greater
Southern Illinois**
140 Iowa Avenue, Suite A
Belleville, IL 62220-3940
(618) 236-2181
FAX: (618) 236-3654
ellenepilepsy@sbcglobal.net

· INDIANA

Epilepsy Foundation of Indiana
3901 W 86th Street, Suite 380
Indianapolis, IN 46268-1799
(317) 876-0600, (800) 526-6618
FAX: (317) 876-0606
1kat@fuse.net

· KENTUCKY

**Epilepsy Foundation of
Kentuckiana**
501 East Broadway, Suite 380
Louisville, KY 40202-1785
(502) 584-8817, (866) 275-1078
FAX: (502) 584-8940
dmcgrath@efky.org

· LOUISIANA

Epilepsy Foundation of Louisiana
3701 Canal Street, Suite H
New Orleans, LA 70119-6101
(504) 486-6326, (800) 960-0587
FAX: (504) 486-8194
epilepsy@bellsouth.net

· MARYLAND

**Epilepsy Foundation of
Chesapeake Region**
8503 LaSalle Road
Towson, MD 21286-5915
(410) 828-7700, (800) 492-2523
lkingham@epilepsy-foundation.org

· MASSACHUSETTS

**Epilepsy Foundation of
Massachusetts and Rhode Island**
540 Gallivan Boulevard, 2nd Floor
Boston, MA 02124-5463
(617) 506-6041, (888) 576-9996
FAX: (617) 506-6047
info@massri.org

· MICHIGAN

Epilepsy Foundation of Michigan
20300 Civic Center Drive, Suite 250
Southfield, MI 48076-4128
(248) 351-7979, (800) 377-6226
FAX: (248) 351-2101
agorelick@epilepsymichigan.org

· MINNESOTA

**Epilepsy Foundation of
Minnesota**
1600 University W, Suite 205
St. Paul, MN 55104-3825
(651) 287-2300, (800) 779-0777
FAX: (651) 287-2325
bloro@efmn.org

· MISSISSIPPI

**Epilepsy Foundation of
Mississippi**
2001 Airport Road N, Suite 307
Jackson, MS 39232-8849
(601) 936-5222, (800) 898-0291
FAX: (601) 939-0824
bethmsepilepsy@bellsouth.net

· MISSOURI

**Epilepsy Foundation of
Kansas and Western Missouri**
6550 Troost Avenue, Suite B
Kansas City, MO 64131-1266
(816) 444-2800, (800) 972-5163
FAX: (816) 444-6777
staylor@efha.org

**Epilepsy Foundation of
St. Louis Region**
7100 Oakland Avenue
St. Louis, MO 63117-1813
(314) 645-6969, (800) 264-6970
FAX: (314) 645-1520
darla@stl-epil.org

• NEW JERSEY

**Epilepsy Foundation of
New Jersey**
429 River View Plaza
Trenton, NJ 08611-3420
(609) 392-4900, (800) 336-5843
FAX: (609) 392-5621
emjefnj@aol.com

• NEW YORK

**Epilepsy Foundation of
Long Island**
506 Stewart Avenue
Garden City, NY 11530-4706
(516) 739-7733, (888) 672-7154
FAX: (516) 739-1860
rdaly@epil.org

Epilepsy Institute
257 Park Avenue, Suite 302
New York, NY 10010-7304
(212) 677-8550
FAX: (212) 677-5825
pconford@epilepsyinstitute.org

**Epilepsy Foundation of
Northeastern New York**
Three Washington Square
Albany, NY 12205-5523
(518) 456-7501, (800) 894-3223
FAX: (518) 452-1282
jgarab@epilepsyneny.com

**Epilepsy Foundation of
Rochester-Syracuse-Binghamton**
1650 South Avenue, Suite 300
Rochester, NY 14620-3926
(585) 442-4430, (800) 724-7930
FAX: (585) 442-6305
d_milliman@epilepsy-uny.org

• NORTH CAROLINA

**Epilepsy Foundation of
North Carolina**
Wake Forest University health
Sciences
Meads Hall, Medical Center
Boulevard
Winston Salem, NC 27157-0001
(336) 716-2320, (800) 451-0694
FAX: (336) 716-6354
pgibson@wfubmc.edu

• OHIO

**Epilepsy Foundation of
Central Ohio**
510 E North Broadway Street,
Suite 400
Columbus, OH 43214-4114
(614) 261-1100, (800) 878-3226
FAX: (614) 261-1248
nbrantner@epilepsy-ohio.org

**Epilepsy Council of
Greater Cincinnati**
895 Central Avenue, Suite 550
Cincinnati, OH 45202-5757
(513) 721-2905
FAX: (513) 721-0799
Kathy.stewart@fuse.net

**Epilepsy Foundation of
Western Ohio**
7523 Brandt Pike
Huber Heights, OH 45424-2382
(937) 233-2500, (800) 360-3296
FAX: (937) 233-5439
jpoppa@ohioepilepsy.org

• PENNSYLVANIA

**Epilepsy Foundation of
Eastern Pennsylvania**
919 Walnut Street, Suite 700
Philadelphia, PA 19107-5237
(215) 629-5003, (800) 887-7165
FAX: (215) 629-4997
efsepa@efsepa.org

**Epilepsy Foundation of
Western/Central Pennsylvania**
1323 Forbes Avenue, Suite 102
Pittsburgh, PA 15219-4725
(412) 261-5880, (800) 361-5885
FAX: (412) 261-5361
jpainter@efwp.org

• PUERTO RICO

**Sociedad Puertorriquena
De Epilepsia**
Hospital Ruiz Soler
Calle Marginal Final
Bayamon, Puerto Rico 00959
(787) 782-6200
FAX: (787) 782-3991
info@sociedadepilepsiapr.org

• SOUTH CAROLINA

**Epilepsy Foundation of
South Carolina**
652 Bush River Road, Suite 211
Columbia, SC 29210-7537
(803) 798-8502
FAX: (803) 798-8591
epilepsysc@epilepsysc.org

• TENNESSEE

**Epilepsy Foundation of
Southeast Tennessee**
744 McCallie Avenue, Suite 517
Chattanooga, TN 37403-2520
(423) 756-1771
FAX: (423) 265-7387
bcoleman@epilepsy-setn.org

**Epilepsy Foundation of
East Tennessee**
1715 E Magnolia Avenue
Knoxville, TN 37917-7827
(865) 522-4991, (800) 522-4991
FAX: (865) 546-5531
lynn@efeasttn.org

Epilepsy Foundation of Middle and West Tennessee
2002 Richard Jones Road, Suite C202
Nashville, TN 37215-2809
(615) 269-7091, (800) 244-0768
FAX: (615) 269-7093
jwhitmer@epilepsytn.org

• **TEXAS**

Epilepsy Foundation of Greater North Texas
8802 Harry Hines Boulevard
Dallas, TX 75235-1716
(214) 823-8809, (888) 548-9716
FAX: (214) 823-8855
dstahlhut@efset.org

Epilepsy Foundation of Southeast Texas
2630 Fountain View, Suite 210
Houston, TX 77057-7629
(713) 789-6295, (888) 548-9716
FAX: (713) 789-5628
dstahlhut@efset.org

Epilepsy Foundation of Central and South Texas
10615 Perrin Beitel Road, Suite 602
San Antonio, TX 78217-3142
(210) 653-5353, (888) 606-5353
FAX: (210) 653-5355
sindi@efcst.org

• **VERMONT**

Epilepsy Foundation of Vermont
P.O. Box 6292
Rutland, VT 05702-6292
(802) 775-1686
FAX: (802) 773-2150
epilepsy@sover.net

• **VIRGINIA**

Epilepsy Foundation of Virginia
P.O. Box 800659
UVA Medical Center
Charlottesville, VA 22908-0659
(434) 924-8669
FAX: (434) 982-6951
srb3m@hscmail.mcc.virginia.edu

• **WASHINGTON**

Epilepsy Foundation of Northwest
3800 Aurora Avenue N, Suite 370
Seattle, WA 98103-8721
(206) 547-4551
FAX: (206) 547-4557
kristacs@epilepsynw.org

• **WEST VIRGINIA**

Epilepsy Foundation of West Virginia
238 4th Avenue, Suite 106
South Charleston, WV 25303-1539
(304) 746-9570, (800) 707-0997
FAX: (304) 746-5554
info@efwv.org

· WISCONSIN

**Epilepsy Foundation of
Southeast Wisconsin**
735 N Water Street, Suite 701
Milwaukee, WI 53202-4104
(414) 271-0110
FAX: (414) 271-0800
epilsew@aol.com

**Epilepsy Foundation of
Western Wisconsin**
1812 Brackett Avenue, Suite 5
Eau Claire, WI 54701-4677
(715) 834-4455, (800) 924-2105
FAX: (715) 834-4465
kbergefww@sbcglobal.net

**Epilepsy Foundation of
South Central Wisconsin**
1302 Mendota Street, Suite 100
Madison, WI 53714-1059
(608) 442-5555, (800) 657-4929
FAX: (608) 442-7474
ataggart@wisc.edu

**Epilepsy Foundation of
Central and Northeast Wisconsin**
1004 First Street, Suite 5
Stevens Point, WI 54481-2627
(715) 341-5811, (800) 924-9932
FAX: (715) 341-5713
cindypiotrowski@efcnw.com

**Epilepsy Foundation of
Southern Wisconsin**
205 North Main Street, Suite 106
Janesville, WI 53545-30625
(608) 755-1821, (800) 693-2287
FAX: (608) 741-0718
jld_efsw@yahoo.com

Comprehensive Epilepsy Centers

· ALABAMA

UAB Epilepsy Center
1719 6th Avenue S
CIRC 312
Birmingham, AL 35294-0021
(205) 934-3866
www.uab.edu/neurology
Medical Director: R. Edward
Faught, MD
Associate Director: Robert
Knowlton, MD

· ARIZONA

**Barrow Neurological Institute
Epilepsy Center**
St. Joseph's Hospital and Medical
Center
350 W Thomas Road
BNI 8th Floor
Phoenix, AZ 85013-4496
(800) 227-7691
www.thebarrow.org/intradoc-cgi/
idc_cgi_isapi.dll?IdcService=SS_GET_
PAGE&nodeId=5012208
Medical Director: David Treiman, MD

**Arizona Comprehensive Epilepsy
Program at University Medical
Center**
1501 N Campbell Avenue
Tucson, AZ 85724
(520) 694-4564
www.neurology.arizona.edu/Clinical/
epilepsy.html
Medical Director: David M.
Labiner, M.D.

**Mayo Clinic Arizona Epilepsy
Center**
Mayo Clinic Hospital
5777 E Mayo Boulevard
Phoenix, AZ 85054
(480) 342-2000
www.mayoclinic.org/epilepsyclinic-sct/
Medical Director: Joseph
Drazkowski, MD

· CALIFORNIA

Loma Linda University Medical Center Comprehensive Epilepsy Center
11234 Anderson Street
MC-A236
Loma Linda, CA 92354
(909) 558-4415
www.llu.edu/llumc/neurosciences/epilepsy.html
Medical Director: Lori Uber Zak, DO, MPT

Cedars-Sinai Epilepsy Program
8700 Beverly Boulevard
North Tower
Room 4127
Los Angeles, CA 90048
(310) 659-7475
www.cedars-sinai.edu/3014.html
Medical Director: Dawn Eliashiv, MD

UCLA Seizure Disorder Center
710 Westwood Plaza
Room 1250
Los Angeles, CA 90095
(310) 825-5745
epilepsy.neurology.ucla.edu
Medical Director: Marc Nuwer, MD, PhD

Hoag Hospital Epilepsy Center
Hoag Memorial Hospital
One Hoag Drive
Newport Beach, CA 92663

(949) 764-8319
www.hoaghospital.org/epilepsy/
Medical Director: Richard Kim, MD, MS

UC Irvine Comprehensive Epilepsy Program
101 The City Drive
Orange, CA 92868
(714) 456-6203
www.ucihealth.com/ep.asp
Program Director: Howard L. Kim, MD

The Epilepsy and Brain Mapping Program
10 Congress Street
Suite 505
Pasadena, CA 91105
(626) 792-7300
www.epipro.com
Medical Director: William W. Sutherling, MD

Sutter NeuroScience Institute Epilepsy Program
2800 L, Suite 500
Sacramento, CA 95816
(916) 733-8338
checksutterfirst.org/neuro/epilepsy/
Medical Director: Robert Burgerman, MD

Sacramento Comprehensive Epilepsy Program
3319 J Street
Sacramento, CA 95816
(916) 325-9101
Medical Director: Robert Burgerman, MD

University of California San Diego Epilepsy Center
UCSD Thornton Hospital
9300 Campus Point Drive
Mail Code 7740
San Diego, CA 92103
(858) 657-6080
health.ucsd.edu/specialties/epilepsy.asp
Medical Director: Vincente J. Iragui, MD, PhD

UCSF Epilepsy Center
University of California San Francisco Medical Center
400 Parnassus Avenue
Box 0138
Room A889
San Francisco, CA 94143-0138
(415) 353-2437
www.ucsfhealth.org/adult/medical_services/neuro/epilepsy/index.html
Medical Director: Daniel H. Lowenstein, MD

Stanford Comprehensive Epilepsy Center
Stanford University
300 Pasteur Drive
Neurology Room A 343
Stanford, CA 94305-5235
(650) 725-6648
www.stanfordhospital.com/clinicsmedServices/COE/neuro/epilepsy/
Medical Director: Robert S. Fisher, MD, PhD

• COLORADO

University of Colorado Hospital Comprehensive Epilepsy Center
University of Colorado Hospital
1635 N Ursula Street
Anschutz Outpatient Pavilion
P.O. Box 6510, Mail Stop F727
Aurora, CO 80045-0510
(720) 848-2080
www.uch.edu/content/epilepsy/content.asp?index=Epilepsy&title=Epilepsy
Medical Director: Mark C. Spitz, MD

CNI (Colorado Neurological Institute) Epilepsy Center
701 E Hampden, Suite 530
Englewood, CO 80113
(303) 788-4600
www.thecni.org/epilepsy/
Medical Director: Barbara Lynne Phillips, MD

• CONNECTICUT

Yale Epilepsy Program
Yale School of Medicine
Yale New Haven Hospital
20 York Street
New Haven, CT 06510
(203) 785-3865
www.epilepsy.yale.edu
Medical Director: Susan Spencer, MD

• FLORIDA

**UF and Shands Comprehensive
Epilepsy Program**
Evelyn F. and William L. McKnight
Brain Institute
Shands Healthcare at UF
1600 SW Archer Road
Box 100-236
Gainesville, FL 32610
(352) 273-5550
www.neurology.ufl.edu/epilepsy/
research.html
Medical Director: Stephan
Eisenschenk, MD

**The Comprehensive Epilepsy
Program at Shands Jacksonville**
UF and Shands
580 W 8th Street
Suite 9, Tower I
Jacksonville, FL 32209
(904) 244-9970
jax.shands.org/hs/neuro/epilepsy.asp
Medical Director: Ramon
Bautista, MD
Comedical Director: Juan Ochoa, MD

**Miami Children's Hospital
Comprehensive Epilepsy Center**
3200 SW 62nd Avenue
Miami, FL 33155
(305) 662-8342
www.mch.com/clinical/neurology.htm
Medical Director: Michael S.
Duchowny, MD

International Center for Epilepsy
Department of Neurology
Miller School of Medicine
1150 NW 14th Street
Suite 410
Miami, FL 33136
(305) 243-5944
Medical Director: R. Eugene
Ramsay, MD

**Bayfront Medical Center
Comprehensive Epilepsy Program**
Bayfront Medical Center
601 7th Street S
St. Petersburg, FL 33701
(727) 553-7923
www.epicareflorida.com
Medical Director: Erasmo A.
Passaro, MD

**Tampa General Hospital and
University of South Florida
Epilepsy Center**
PO Box 1289
Tampa, FL 33601-1289
(813) 844-4675
epilepsy.usf.edu
Medical Director: Selim Benbadis, MD

University Community Hospital, Inc.
Neurodiagnostics Epilepsy Program
3100 E Fletcher Avenue
Tampa, FL 33613
(813) 615-7279
Medical Director: Paul Winters, MD
Comedical Director: Nancy
Rodgers-Neame, MD

· GEORGIA

Emory University Epilepsy Center
Department of Neurology
101 Woodruff Circle, Suite 6000
Atlanta, GA 30322
(404) 778-5943
www.emoryhealthcare.org/
departments/epilepsy/index.html
Medical Director: Page Pennell, MD

Children's Epilepsy Center
Children's Healthcare of Atlanta at
Scottish Rite
1001 Johnson Ferry Road NE
Atlanta, GA 30342
(800) 803-5437, (404) 785-2186
www.choa.org/default.aspx?ID=869
Medical Director: J. Robert
Flamini, MD
Surgical Director: Roger Hudgins, MD

Piedmont Hospital Epilepsy Center
1968 Peachtree Road NW
Atlanta, GA 30309

(404) 605-3244, (404) 351-2270
www.piedmont.org,
www.peachtreeneurological.com
Medical Director: Lawrence G.
Seiden, MD

MCG Comprehensive Epilepsy Program
Medical College of Georgia
1120 15th Street
Augusta, GA 30912
(706) 721-4626
www.mcgepilepsy.com
Medical Director: Yong Park, MD

The Georgia Neuro Center
The Medical Center of Central
Georgia
777 Hemlock Street
HBO 34
Macon, GA 31208
(478) 633-1184
www.mccg.org/services/neuro.asp
Medical Director: Erich Richter, MD

· HAWAII

The Queen's Epilepsy Center
The Queen's Medical Center
1301 Punchbowl Street
Honolulu, HI 96813
(808) 585-5494
www.queens.org/services/
neuroscience.html
Medical Director: Alan Stein, MD

• IOWA

Iowa Comprehensive Epilepsy Program
Department of Neurology
200 Hawkins Drive
Iowa City, IA 52242
(319) 356-7235
www.uihealthcare.com/depts/med/
neurology/patients/epilepsyprogram/
index.html
Medical Director: Mark Granner, MD

• IDAHO

Idaho Comprehensive Epilepsy Center
Consultants in Epilepsy and
Neurology, PLLC
190 E. Bannock
Boise, ID 83712
(208) 381-7353
www.stlukesonline.org/boise/
specialties_and_services/epilepsy/
Medical Director: Robert T. Wechsler,
MD, PhD

• ILLINOIS

The University of Chicago Hospitals Adult Epilepsy Center
The University of Chicago
5841 S Maryland Avenue
Mail Code 2030
Chicago, IL 60637
(773) 834-4703
www.uchospitals.edu/specialties/
epilepsy/

Medical Director: John S.
Ebersole, MD
Comedical Director: James X Tao,
MD, PhD

Rush Epilepsy Center
Rush University Medical Center
1653 W Congress Parkway
Chicago, IL 60612
(312) 942-5939
www.rush.edu/rumc/
page-1099611538227.html
Medical Director: Michael C.
Smith, MD

Northwestern University Comprehensive Epilepsy Center
251 E Huron 7-104
Attn: Emma Cook
Chicago, IL 60611
(312) 926-1673
www.feinberg.northwestern.edu/
depts/neurology/index.html
Medical Director: Stephan Schuele
MD, MPH
Comedical Director: Prashanthi
Boppana, MD

University of Chicago Pediatric Epilepsy Center
University of Chicago Comer
Children's Hospital
5721 S Maryland Avenue
MC 3055
Chicago, IL 60637
(773) 702-6487

www.uchicagokidshospital.org/
specialties/epilepsy
Medical Director: David Frim,
MD, PhD
Comedical Director: Michael
Kohrman, MD

**Loyola University Medical Center
Comprehensive Epilepsy Program**
2160 S First Avenue
Maywood, IL 60153
(708) 216-9000
www.luhs.org/svcline/neuro/services/
epilepsy.htm
Medical Director: Jorge Asconape, MD

· INDIANA

**Indiana University
Comprehensive Epilepsy Program**
University Hospital
550 N University Boulevard
UH Room 1711
Indianapolis, IN 46202
(317) 274-4974
indianaepilepsyservices.iusm.iu.edu/
iucomprehensiveepilepsycenter.htm
Medical Director: Vincenta
Salanova, MD

· KANSAS

**Via Christi Comprehensive
Epilepsy Center**
848 N St Francis
Suite 3950
Wichita, KS 67214
(316) 268-8500

www.via-christi.org/epilepsy
Medical Director: Kore K. Liow, MD

· KENTUCKY

**UK Comprehensive Epilepsy
Center**
University of KY Chandler Medical
Center
740 S Limestone-KY Clinic
Room L-445
Lexington, KY 40536-0284
(859) 257-7591
ukhealthcare.uky.edu/KNI/
clinic_epilepsy.htm
Medical Director: Toufic Fakhoury,
MD

**University of Louisville
Comprehensive Epilepsy Center**
Epilepsy Monitoring Unit
530 S Jackson Street
Louisville, KY 40202
(502) 562-4169
www.uoflhealthcare.org/
MoreProgramsServices/
ComprehensiveEpilepsyCenter/
tabid/305/Default.aspx
Medical Director: Pradeep Modur, MD

· MARYLAND

**University of Maryland Epilepsy
Center**
22 S Greene Street
Room N4W46
Baltimore, MD 21201
(410) 328-6266

www.umm.edu/neurosciences/
epilepsycenter.html
Medical Director: Allan Krumholz, MD
Epilepsy Monitoring Unit Director:
Jennifer Hopp, MD

Johns Hopkins Epilepsy Center
600 N Wolfe Street
Meyer 2-147
Baltimore, MD 21287
(410) 955-7338
www.hopkinsneuro.org/epilepsy/
Medical Director: Gregory K.
Bergey, MD

· MASSACHUSETTS

**Beth Israel Deaconess Epilepsy
Program**
Beth Israel Deaconess Medical Center
Harvard Medical School
330 Brookline Avenue
504 Baker Building
Boston, MA 02215
(617) 632-8930
www.bidmc.harvard.edu/display.
asp?node_id=7984
Medical Director: Donald Schomer, MD

**Children's Hospital Boston
Comprehensive Epilepsy Center**
300 Longwood Avenue
Fegan 9
Boston, MA 02115
(617) 355-2413
www.childrenshospital.
org/clinicalservices/Site1549/
mainpageS1549P0.html

Medical Director: Blaise
Bourgeois, MD

MGH Epilepsy Center
55 Fruit Street
WAC 720
Boston, MA 02114
(617) 726-3311
www.seizure.org
Medical Director: Andrew Cole,
MD, FRCP (c)

**Boston Medical Center Epilepsy
Care Program for Children and
Adults**
One Boston Medical Center Place
Boston, MA 02118
(617) 414-1099
www.bmc.org
Medical Director: Georgia
Montouris, MD
Comedical Director: Thomas R.
Browne, MD

BWH Epilepsy Center
Brigham and Women's Hospital
75 Francis Street
Tower 5-D
Boston, MA 02115
(617) 732-7547
www.brighamandwomens.org/
neurology/epilepsy/epilepsyteam.aspx
Medical Director: Barbara
Dworetzky, MD
Comedical Director: Peter M.
Black, MD

Lahey Clinic Epilepsy Center
41 Mall Road
Burlington, MA 01805
(781) 744-8665
www.lahey.org/neurology/
neurology_seizuresepilepsy.asp
Medical Director: Joel Oster, MD

- MICHIGAN

University of Michigan Comprehensive Epilepsy Program
1500 E Medical Center Drive
lB300 UH-0036
Ann Arbor, MI 48109-0036
(734) 936-9030
www.med.umich.edu/neuro/epilepsy
Medical Director: Linda Selwa, MD

Henry Ford Health System Comprehensive Epilepsy Program
Department of Neurology, K-11
Henry Ford Hospital
2799 W Grand Boulevard
Detroit, MI 48202
(313) 916-2451
www.henryford.com/body.
cfm?id=45102
Medical Director: Brien Smith, MD

Wayne State University/Detroit Medical Center
Comprehensive Epilepsy Program
Harper University Hospital/Wayne
State University
4201 St Antoine

8D-University Health Center
Detroit, MI 48201-2153
(313) 745-1416
www.med.wayne.edu/neurology/clin_
programs/Labs/Epilepsy/epilepsy.html
Medical Director: Craig Watson,
MD, PhD

- MINNESOTA

MINCEP Epilepsy Care
5775 Wayzata Boulevard, Suite 200
Minneapolis, MN 55416
(952) 525-2400
www.mincep.com
Medical Director: Robert J.
Gumnit, MD

Mayo Clinic Foundation Epilepsy Center
200 First Street SW
Rochester, MN 55905
(507) 538-1032
www.mayoclinic.org/epilepsy/
Medical Director: Gregory D.
Cascino, MD

Minnesota Epilepsy Group, PA® of United and Children's Hospitals and Clinics of Minnesota–St. Paul
225 Smith Avenue N, Suite 201
St. Paul, MN 55102
(651) 241-5290
www.mnepilepsy.org
Medical Director: Michael D.
Frost, MD

• MISSISSIPPI

University of Mississippi Medical Center Epilepsy Program
Department of Neurology
2500 N State Street
Jackson, MS 39216
(601) 984-4760
neurology.umc.edu/index.
php?d=cs&p=epilepsy
Medical Director: Mecheri
Sundaram, MD

• MISSOURI

The Comprehensive Epilepsy Care Center for Children and Adults
St. Luke's Hospital
222 S Woods Mill Road
Suite 610 N
Chesterfield, MO 63017
(314) 453-9300
Medical Director: William
Rosenfield, MD
Comedical Director: Susan
Lippmann, MD

Comprehensive Epilepsy Center
St. Luke's Brain and Stroke Institute
St. Luke's Hospital
4401 Wornall Road
Kansas City, MO 64111
(816) 932-6002
www.saintlukeshealthsystem.org/
slhs/locations/saint_lukes_brain_
and_stroke_institute/(pf)overview.htm
Medical Director: John E.
Croom, MD, PhD

Epilepsy Centers at Washington University
Pediatric Epilepsy Center
St. Louis Children's Hospital
One Children's Place, Suite 12E47
(Admin)
St. Louis, MO 63110-1093
(314) 454-4089
www.peds.wustl.edu/clinical/
epilepsy.html
Medical Director: Liu-Lin
Thio, MD, PhD

Washington University Comprehensive Department of Epilepsy
Barnes Jewish Hospital
Box 8111
660 S Euclid Avenue
St. Louis, MO 63110
(314) 362-7845
www.neuro.wustl.edu/epilepsy/adult
Medical Director: R. Edward
Hogan, MD

• MONTANA

Montana Epilepsy Program
Benefis Healthcare
500 15th Avenue South
Great Falls, MT 59405
(406) 455-2800
www.benefis.org/pages/default.
asp?NavID=122
Medical Director: Bradley Davis, MD

· NEBRASKA

Immanuel Medical Center
Epilepsy Care Center
6901 N. 72nd Street
Omaha, NE 68122
(422) 572-2566
www.nebraskamed.com/services/
neuro/epilepsy_center/
Medical Director: Richard V.
Andrews, MD

The Nebraska Epilepsy Center
982045 Nebraska Medical Center
Omaha, NE 68198-2045
(402) 559-3939
www.nebraskamed.com/services/
neuro/nebraska_epilepsy_center/
default.aspx
Medical Director: Sanjay P.
Singh, MD

· NEW MEXICO

Comprehensive Epilepsy Center
of New Mexico
University of New Mexico
2211 Lomas Bloulevard
NE ACC 2nd Floor
Albuquerque, NM 87106
(505) 272-3342
hsc.unm.edu/som/bmb/Signature%
20Research%20Prgms/brain_and_
behaviorial.shtml
Medical Director: Bruce Fisch, MD

· NEW JERSEY

Pediatric Neuroscience Institute
and Comprehensive Epilepsy
Center
Hackensack University Medical
Center
20 Prospect Avenue, Suite 800
Hackensack, NJ 07601
(201) 996-3200
www.humc.com/pediatricneurology/
Medical Director: Marcelo E.
Lancman, MD

Atlantic Neuroscience Institute
Epilepsy Center
Overlook Hospital
99 Beauvoir Avenue
Summit, NJ 07902
(908) 522-4990
www.atlantichealth.org/en/
neuroscience/services/atlantic+neuros
cience+institute's+epilepsy+center/
Medical Director: Marcelo E.
Lancman, MD

· NEW YORK

Albany Medical Center
Comprehensive Epilepsy Center
47 New Scotland Avenue
Albany, NY 12208
(518) 262-5226
www.amc.edu/Patient/services/
Neurosciences/epilepsy/index.html
Medical Director: Anthony L.
Ritaccio, MD

**Montefiore Comprehensive
Epilepsy Management Center**
Albert Einstein College of Medicine
Montefiore Medical Center
111 E 210th Street
Bronx, NY 10467
(718) 920-4378
www.montekids.org/services/
leadership/neurology/epilepsy/
Medical Director: Shlomo
Shinnar, MD
Director of Clinical Neurophysiology:
Solomon Moshe, MD

**NYU Comprehensive Epilepsy
Center**
New York University Hospital Center
403 E 34th Street, 4th Floor
New York, NY 10016
(212) 263-8871
www.nyuepilepsy.org/cec/
Medical Director: Orrin
Devinsky, MD
Comedical Director: Ruben
Kuzniecky, MD

**Weill Cornell Medical Center
Comprehensive Epilepsy Center**
525 E. 68th Street
K-619
New York, NY 10021
(212) 746-2359
www.cornellepilepsy.com
Medical Director: Douglas Labar,
MD, PhD

Strong Epilepsy Center
Strong Memorial Hospital
University of Rochester Medical
Center
601 Elmwood Avenue
Box 673
Rochester, NY 14642
(585) 341-7420
www.stronghealth.com/services/
neurology/epilepsy/
Medical Director: Michel J. Berg, MD
Program Director: Robert Gross,
MD, PhD

SUNY Upstate Medical University
750 E Adams Street
Syracuse, NY 13210
(315) 464-4243
www.upstate.edu/uh/neurology/
epilepsy.php
Medical Director: Robert Beach, MD

· NORTH CAROLINA

**University of North Carolina
Epilepsy Center**
Department of Neurology
University of North Carolina at
Chapel Hill
3100 Bioinformatics Bldg
CB 7025
Chapel Hill, NC 27599
(919) 966-8160
nerve.neurology.unc.edu/neurology/
epilepsy.htm
Medical Director: Robert S.
Greenwood, MD

**Duke University Hospital
Epilepsy Center**
Duke Hospital
Box 2921
Durham, NC 27710
(919) 681-5363
neurology.mc.duke.edu/Epilepsy_
Central_Neurophysiolo.29.0.html
Medical Director: Rodney A.
Radtke, MD

**Wake Forest University
Comprehensive Epilepsy Center**
Baptist Medical Center
Medical Center Boulevard
Winston-Salem, NC 27157
(336) 713-9389
www1.wfubmc.edu/neurology/
Neurology+Sections/Epilepsy/
Clinic.htm
Medical Director: William L. Bell, MD

· OHIO

The Cincinnati Epilepsy Center
The Neuroscience Institute
The University Hospital
234 Goodman
ML 0724
Cincinnati, OH 45219-0724
(513) 584-2214
www.leadingtheadvance.com
Medical Director: Michael
Privitera, MD

**Cleveland Clinic Pediatric
Epilepsy Program**
9500 Euclid Avenue
Cleveland, OH 44195
(216) 444-2200
cms.clevelandclinic.org/neuroscience/
body.cfm?id=126
Medical Director: Elaine Wyllie, MD

**University Hospitals of Cleveland
Comprehensive Epilepsy
Program**
11100 Euclid Avenue
LKSD 3200
Cleveland, OH 44106
(216) 844-3717
www.epilepsy.uhhs.com
Medical Director: Hans Luders,
MD, PhD
Comedical Director: Mark Scher, MD

Cleveland Clinic Epilepsy Center
Cleveland Clinic
9500 Euclid Avenue
S51
Cleveland, OH 44195
(216) 445-5559
www.clevelandclinic.org/epilepsy
Medical Director: Imad Najm, MD

Ohio State University
Comprehensive Epilepsy
Program
1654 Upham Drive
4th Floor—Attn: Dr. Moore
Columbus, OH 43210
(614) 293-4882
medicalcenter.osu.edu/patientcare/
healthcare_services/epilepsy/
Medical Director: J. Layne Moore,
MD, MPH

Mount Carmel Epilepsy Center
793 W State Street
Columbus, OH 43222
(614) 234-5000
www.mountcarmelhealth.com/155.cfm
Medical Director: Jean Cibula, MD
Comedical Director: Denise
Cambier, MD

Comprehensive Epilepsy
Program at Ohio State University
Children's Hospital
700 Children's Drive
Columbus, OH 43205
(614) 722-4600
www.columbuschildrens.
com/GD/Templates/Pages/
Childrens/NeuroSciences/
NeuroSciencesLongContent.aspx?
page=4942&ShowFlash=1
Medical Director: Julian M. Paolicchi,
MA, MD

Riverside Hospital Epilepsy Center
3535 Olentangy River Road
Columbus, OH 43214
(614) 566-4162
www.ohiohealth.com/riversideneuro.
cfm?id=1806
Medical Director: Charles W. Hall, MD
Comedical Director: Denise
Cambier, MD

· OKLAHOMA

Comprehensive Oklahoma
Program for Epilepsy (COPE)
OU Medical Center-Presbyterian
Tower
700 NE 13th Street
Box 31
Oklahoma City, OK 73104
(405) 271-4334
www.oumedcenter.com
Medical Director: K.J. Oommen, MD

· OREGON

OHSU Comprehensive Epilepsy
Center
Oregon Health and Science
University
3181 SW Sam Jackson Park Road
Mail Code L444
Portland, OR 97239
(503) 494-5682
www.ohsu.edu/epilepsy
Medical Director: Martin
Salinsky, MD
Comedical Director: David
Spencer, MD

Providence Epilepsy Center
Providence St Vincent Medical Center
9205 SW Barnes Road
Portland, OR 97225
(503) 291-5300
www.providence.org/oregon/
programs_and_services/brain/
epilepsy/e01default.htm
Medical Director: Mark Yerby, MD

• PENNSYLVANIA

The Penn State Milton S. Hershey Medical Center Comprehensive Epilepsy Center
500 University Drive
H037
Hershey, PA 17033
(717) 531-5600
www.hmc.psu.edu/neurology/
aservices/epilepsy.htm
Medical Director: Paul H.
McCabe, MD
Comedical Director: Matthew
Eccher, MD

Jefferson Comprehensive Epilepsy Center
Thomas Jefferson University
900 Walnut Street, Suite 200
Philadelphia, PA 19107
(215) 955-1222
www.jeffersonhospital.org/
neuroscience/article4319.html
Medical Director: Michael R.
Sperling, MD

Penn Epilepsy Center
University of Pennsylvania
3400 Spruce Street
3 W Gates
Philadelphia, PA 19104-4283
(215) 349-5166
pennhealth.com/neuro/services/
epilepsy/index.html
Medical Director: Peter Crino,
MD, PhD

Allegheny General Hospital Comprehensive Epilepsy Program
420 E North Avenue
Suite 206
Pittsburgh, PA 15212
(412) 359-8850
www.aghneuroscience.com/index.cfm
Medical Director: James P.
Valeriano, MD

University of Pittsburgh Comprehensive Epilepsy Center
3471 5th Avenue
811 Kaufmann Medical Building
Pittsburgh, PA 15213
(412) 692-4609
www.neurosurgery.pitt.edu/epilepsy/
index.html
Medical Director: Anto Bagic, MD
Comedical Director: Patricia
Crumrine, MD

Wellspan Epilepsy Center
290 St Charles Way
York, PA 17405
(717) 851-4585
www.wellspan.org/body.cfm?id=68
Medical Director: Allen E. Tyler, MD

Drexel Epilepsy
Hahnemann Hospital
Broad and Vine Streets
MS 308
Philadelphia, PA 19107-1192
(215) 762-7037
Medical Director: Sigmund
Jenssen, MD

· RHODE ISLAND

**Rhode Island Hospital
Comprehensive Epilepsy
Program**
110 Lockwood Street, POB, Suite 342
Providence, RI 02903
(401) 444-4364
www.lifespan.org/rih/services/
neuro/epilepsy/
Medical Director: Andrew S. Blum,
MD, PhD
Comedical Director: David E.
Mandelbaum, MD, PhD
Surgical Director: John A. Duncan,
III, MD, PhD

· SOUTH CAROLINA

**Medical University of South
Carolina Comprehensive Epilepsy
Center**
96 Jonathan Lucas Street
Charleston, SC 29425
(843) 792-3263
www.muschealth.com/neurosciences/
epilepsy.htm
Medical Director: Jonathan C.
Edwards, MD

· TENNESSEE

**LeBonheur Comprehensive
Epilepsy Program**
LeBonheur Children's Medical Center
50 N Dunlap
Memphis, TN 38103
(888) 890-0818
www.lebonheur.org/portal/site/
lebonheur/menuitem.d2c2a3536e
17341bd11fafd511b18a0c/?
vgnextoid=4b9279e183f1b010Vgn
VCM1000000516a8c0RCRD&
vgnextfmt=default
Medical Director: James W.
Wheless, MD

**Methodist University Hospital
Comprehensive Epilepsy Center**
1265 Union Avenue
Memphis, TN 38104
(901) 516-7478
neuro.methodisthealth.org

Medical Director: Tulio E. Bertorini, MD
Comedical Director: Gregory J. Condon, MD

Vanderbilt University Epilepsy Program
Vanderbilt University Medical Center
A-0118 Medical Center N
Nashville, TN 37232-2551
www.mc.vanderbilt.edu/neurology/epilepsy.htm
Medical Director: Bassel Abou-Khalil, MD

· TEXAS

UT Southwestern Epilepsy Center
Parkland Memorial Hospital and
Children's Medical Center of Dallas
5201 Harry Hines Boulevard
8th Floor
Dallas, TX 75235
(214) 590-8340
www8.utsouthwestern.edu/utsw/cda/dept14431/files/81593.html
Medical Directors: Paul C. Van Ness, MD (adult) and Susan Arnold, MD (pediatric)

Medical City Center for Epilepsy
Medical City Dallas Hospital
7777 Forest Lane
Dallas, TX 75230
(972) 566-4223

www.medicalcityhospital.com/customPage.asp?PageName=Epilepsy_Home
Medical Director: Robert Leroy, MD

Texas Epilepsy Group
Presbyterian Hospital of Dallas
8200 Walnut Hill Lane, Jackson 2 West
Dallas, TX 75231
(214) 345-4155
www.texashealth.org
Medical Director: Jay H. Harvey, DO

Cook Children's Comprehensive Epilepsy Program
Department of Child Neurology
Cook Children's Medical Center
901 Seventh Avenue
Suite 120
Fort Worth, TX 76104
(682) 885-2500
www.cookchildrens.org/
Medical Director: Angel W. Hernandez, MD

The Comprehensive Texas Regional Epilepsy Center (C-TREC)
301 University Blvd
9.128 John Sealy Annex
Galveston, TX 77555-0539
(409) 772-2646
Medical Director: Joseph A. Oommen, MD

Baylor Comprehensive Epilepsy Center at St. Luke's Episcopal Hospital
Department of Neurology-NB 302
Baylor College of Medicine/St. Luke's Episcopal Hospital
One Baylor Plaza
Houston, TX 77030
(713) 798-0980
www.BaylorEpilepsyCenter.org
Medical Director: Eli M. Mizrahi, MD

Texas Comprehensive Epilepsy Program
University of Texas at Houston
6431 Fannin
MSB 7 104
Houston, TX 77030
(713) 500-7117
www.texasepilepsycenter.com
Medical Director: Jeremy Slater, MD

South Texas Comprehensive Epilepsy Center
NeuroDiagnostic Center
UTHSCSA/University Hospital/AMVAH
4502 Medical Drive
San Antonio, TX 78229
(218) 358-2310
www.texasepilepsy.net
Medical Director: Charles Akos Szabo, MD

· UTAH

University of Utah Comprehensive Epilepsy Program
Department of Neurology
3R210 SOM, 30 N 1900 E
Salt Lake City, UT 84132
(801) 585-6387
healthcare.utah.edu/medicalServices/index.cfm?fuseaction=controller.getDivision&divisionKey=34
Medical Director: Tawnya Constantino, MD

· VIRGINIA

FE Dreifuss Comprehensive Epilepsy Program
University of Virginia Health Systems
Hospital Drive
PO Box 800394
McKim Hall, Room 2027
Charlottesville, VA 22908
(434) 924-5312
www.UVAepilepsy.com
Medical Director: Nathan Fountain, MD

Epilepsy Institute of Virginia
Department of Neurology
Virginia Commonwealth University
Box 980599
Richmond, VA 23298-0599
(804) 828-0442
Medical Director: John M. Pellock, MD
Comedical Director: Lawrence Morton, PhD

· WASHINGTON

WA Neuroscience Institute at Valley Medical Center
Valley Professional Center N
3915 Talbot Road S
Suite 104
Renton, WA 98055
(425) 656-5566
www.waneuro.org
Medical Director: David Vossler, MD

Swedish Epilepsy Center
Seattle Neuroscience Institute
801 Broadway
Suite 901
Seattle, WA 98122
(206) 386-3880
www.swedish.org/body.
cfm?id=22&oTopID=22
Medical Director: Michael
Doherty, MD

UW Regional Epilepsy Center
325 Ninth Avenue
Box 359745
Seattle, WA 98104
(206) 731-3576
pcs.hmc.washington.edu/Epilepsy/
Index.htm
Medical Director: John W.
Miller, MD, PhD

· WEST VIRGINIA

West Virginia University Hospitals Epilepsy Center
West Virginia Hospitals
PO Box 8202
One Stadium Drive
Morgantown, WV 26506-9180
304-598-4330
www.hsc.wvu.edu/som/neurology/
seizureSurgeryProgram.asp
Medical Director: Adrianna
Palade, MD
Comedical Director: Warren
Boling, MD

· WISCONSIN

Marshfield Clinic
1000 N Oak Avenue
Marshfield, WI 54449-5777
(715) 387-5511, (800) 699-3377
www.marshfieldclinic.org/patients/
default.aspx?page=neuro_
specialties_epilepsy
Medical Director: Evan Sandok, MD

Medical College of Wisconsin Adult Epilepsy Center
8701 Watertown Plank Road
Milwaukee, WI 53226
(414) 805-5206
www.mcw.edu/display/router.
asp?docid=13550
Medical Director: Manoj
Raghavan, MD

Medical College of Wisconsin
Pediatric Epilepsy Center
8701 Watertown Plank Road
Milwaukee, WI 53226
(414) 266-3464
www.mcw.edu/display/router.
asp?docid=2022
Medical Director: Mary Zupanc, MD

• WYOMING

Wyoming Epilepsy Center
1233 E 2nd Street
Casper, WY 82601
(307) 577-2225
www.wyomingneurology.com/
epilepsy.htm
Medical Director: David B. Wheeler,
MD, PhD

Driving and Epilepsy*

STATE	SEIZURE-FREE PERIOD	PHYSICIANS MUST REPORT?
Alabama	6 months	no
Alaska	6 months	no
Arizona	3 months	no
Arkansas	1 year	no
California	not set	yes
Colorado	not set	no
Connecticut	not set	no
Delaware	not set	yes
District of Columbia	1 year	no
Florida	not set	no
Georgia	6 months	no
Hawaii	6 months	no
Idaho	6 months	no
Illinois	not set	no
Indiana	not set	no
Iowa	6 months	no
Kansas	6 months	no
Kentucky	3 months	no
Louisiana	6 months	no

*Updated August, 1, 2007.

Maine	3 months	no
Maryland	not set	no
Massachusetts	6 months	no
Michigan	6 months	no
Minnesota	6 months	no
Mississippi	1 year	no
Missouri	6 months	no
Montana	not set	no
Nebraska	3 months	no
Nevada	3 months	yes
New Hampshire	1 year	no
New Jersey	1 year	yes
New Mexico	1 year	no
New York	1 year	no
North Carolina	6–12 months	no
North Dakota	6 months	no
Ohio	not set	no
Oklahoma	6 months	no
Oregon	6 months	yes
Pennsylvania	6 months	yes
Puerto Rico	not set	no
Rhode Island	18 months	no
South Carolina	6 months	no
South Dakota	6–12 months	no
Tennessee	6 months	no
Texas	6 months	no
Utah	3 months	no
Vermont	not set	no
Virginia	6 months	no
Washington	6 months	no
West Virginia	1 year	no
Wisconsin	3 months	no
Wyoming	3 months	no

F

Epilepsy Summer Camps

For information about scholarships, contact the
Epilepsy Foundation (800) 332-1000.

· ALABAMA

The Epilepsy Foundation of
South Alabama and the Epilepsy
Foundation of North/Central
Alabama
Camp Candlelight at Camp ASCCA
Ages: 6–18
(800) 626-1582
(251) 432-0970
dtoenes@epilepsysouthalabama.org

· ARIZONA

Epilepsy Foundation of Arizona
Camp Candlelight
Ages: 8–15
(888) 768-2690
(602) 406-3581

· CALIFORNIA

The Epilepsy Foundation of
Greater Los Angeles
Teen Retreat
Ages: 12–19
(310) 670-2870

Family Camp
Ages: 5–20, parents, siblings
(310) 670-2870

Epilepsy Foundation of
Northern California
Camp Coelho
Ages: 9–15
williams@epilepsynorcal.org

Epilepsy Foundation of
San Diego County
Camp Quest
Ages: 8–12
(619) 296-0161

· COLORADO

Epilepsy Foundation of Colorado
Jason Fleishman Summer Camp
Ages: 10–17
(303) 377-9774

· CONNECTICUT

Epilepsy Foundation of Connecticut
Summer Camp for Children with Epilepsy
Ages: 6–18
(800) 899-3745
efct@sbcglobal.net
www.epilepsyct.net

· FLORIDA

Epilepsy Foundation of Florida
Camp Boggy Creek
Ages: 7–16
www.BoggyCreek.org, www.epilepsyfla.org

· GEORGIA

Epilepsy Foundation of Georgia
Camp Lakewood
Ages: 8–18
Camp Big Heart
Ages: 8–21
Ages: 21+
(800) 527-7105

· HAWAII

Epilepsy Foundation of Hawaii
Camp Kukui
Ages: 6–18
(808) 528-3058
EFH@Hawaiiepilepsy.com

· ILLINOIS

The Epilepsy Foundation of Greater Chicago
Camp Blackhawk
Ages: 6–18
(312) 939-8622

· KANSAS AND MISSOURI

Epilepsy Foundation of Kansas and Western Missouri
Camp Shing
Ages: 6–17, parents, siblings
(800) 972-5163
(816) 444-2800

· LOUISIANA

The Epilepsy Foundation of Louisiana
Camp Alabama
Ages: 6–16
(800) 960-0587
(877) 282-0802
caleb@medcamps.com

• MARYLAND

**Epilepsy Foundation of the
Chesapeake Region**
Camp Great Rock
Ages: 7–16
(202) 884-5142

• MASSACHUSETTS AND
  RHODE ISLAND

**Epilepsy Foundation of
Massachusetts and Rhode Island**
Camp Wee-Kan-Tu
Ages: 8–17
(617) 506-6041
sdagen@partners.org

• MICHIGAN

Epilepsy Foundation of Michigan
Camp Discovery
Ages: Grades 3–10
(800) 377-6226 xt.1-231
sdarroch@epilepsymichigan.org

• MINNESOTA

**Epilepsy Foundation of
Minnesota**
Camp OZ
Ages: 9–17
(800) 779-0777, ext. 2308
(651) 287-2308
nbaker@efmn.org
www.efmn.org

• MISSISSIPPI

**Epilepsy Foundation of
Mississippi**
Alvin P. Flannes Summer Camp
Ages: 8–16
(800) 898-0291
(601) 936-5222
phymsepilepsy@bellsouth.net

• NEW JERSEY

**Epilepsy Foundation of
New Jersey**
Camp NOVA
Ages: 12–28
(856) 858-5900
hsherman@efnj.com

**Mighty Mike's Bounce Out the
Stigma Basketball Camp in
Conjunction with the Epilepsy
Foundation of New Jersey**
Ages: 9–18
(201) 725-7224
(973) 244-0850
www.bounceoutthestigma.com

• NEW YORK

**Epilepsy Foundation of
Northeastern New York, Inc.**
Ages: 5–18
(518) 456-7501
dbain@epilepsyneny.com

**Epilepsy Foundation of
Rochester, Syracuse, Binghamton**
Camp EAGR
Ages: 8–15
(585) 442-4430, ext. 2702
m_radell@epilepsy-uny.org

• NORTH CAROLINA

**Epilepsy Foundation of
North Carolina**
Camp Carefree
Ages: 6–16
(336) 427-0966
www.campcarefree.org

Victory Junction Gang Camp
Ages: 7–15
(336) 498-9055
www.victoryjunction.org

• OHIO

**Epilepsy Foundation of Central
Ohio and Epilepsy Foundation of
Western Ohio**
Camp Firebird
Ages: 7–17
(800) 878-3226
(614) 261-1100
kbrown@epilepsy-ohio.org
www.epilepsy-ohio.org

**Epilepsy Foundation of Greater
Cincinnati and the Epilepsy
Foundation of Kentuckiana**
Camp Dream Catcher
Ages: 8+
(877) 804-2241
www.epilepsyfoundation.org/
cincinnati

• PENNSYLVANIA

**Epilepsy Foundation of Eastern
Pennsylvania**
Camp Achieve
Ages: preteens and teens
(215) 629-5003

**Epilepsy Foundation of
Western/Central Pennsylvania**
Camp Frog
Ages: 8–17
Camp Fitch: (800) 361-5885
kwilson@efwp.org
Camp Conrad Weiser: (800) 336-0301
gknaub@efwp.org

• SOUTH CAROLINA

**Epilepsy Foundation of
South Carolina**
Camp River Run
Ages: 7–14
(803) 798-8502
www.epilepsysc.org

· TENNESSEE

**Epilepsy Foundation of East
Tennessee and the Epilepsy
Foundation of Middle and West
Tennessee**
Camp Discovery
Ages: 7–19 and older
(800) 951-4991
(865) 522-4991

· TEXAS

**Epilepsy Foundation of
Southeast Texas**
Camp Spike'n'Wave
Ages: 8–14
(888) 548-9716
(713) 789-6295
MTrotter@efset.org

Camp Kaleidoscope
Ages: 15–19
(888) 548-9716
(713) 789-6295
MTrotter@efset.org

· VIRGINIA

Epilepsy Foundation of Virginia
Ages: 9–13
(757) 438-2398
www.efvase.org

· WASHINGTON

Epilepsy Foundation Northwest
Camp discovery
Ages: 7–17
(800) 752-3509
ahancock@epilepsynw.org
www.epilepsynw.org

· WISCONSIN

Camp Phoenix
Ages: 8–17
Epilepsy Foundation Central and
Northwest Wisconsin (800) 924-9932
Epilepsy Foundation South Central
Wisconsin (800) 657-4929
Epilepsy Foundation Southeast
Wisconsin (414) 271-0110
Epilepsy Foundation Southern
Wisconsin (800) 693-2287
Epilepsy Foundation Western
Wisconsin (800) 924-2105

G

International Epilepsy Resources

Member List for the International Bureau for Epilepsy

· ARGENTINA

Asociacion de Lucha contra
la Epilepsia
Tucuman 3261
1189 Buenos Aires
+54 114 8620 440
FAX: +54 114 862 0440
gonzalezgartland@aol.com

· AUSTRALIA

Joint Epilepsy Council of
Australia Limited (JECA)
818 Burke Road
Camberwell
Vic 3124
Australia
+61 3 9805 9111
FAX: +61 3 9882 7159

· AUSTRIA

Epilepsie Dachverband
Österreich
Wichtelgasse 55/17–19
1170 Wien
Austria
+43 1 489 52 78
FAX: +43 1 489 60 51
epilepsie@aon.at
www.epilepsie.at

· BANGLADESH

Epilepsy Association of
Bangladesh
3/1 Lake Circus
Kalabagan
Dhaka 1205
Bangladesh
+88 02 811 4846
FAX: +88 02 812 4351
neurologyfoundation@yahoo.com
www.neurologyfoundation.org

· BELGIUM

**Les Amis de la Ligue Nationale
Belge contre l'Epilepsie**
Avenue Albert 135
Brussels 1190
Belgium
+32 2344 3263
FAX: +32 2343 6837
epilepsy.belgium@skynet.be

· BRAZIL

**Associacao Brasileira de
Epilepsia**
R Botucatu 740
CEP 04023–900
Sao Paulo, SP
Brazil
+55 11 55 49 3819
abe@epilepsiabrasil.org.br
www.epilepsiabrasil.org.br

· BULGARIA

**Association for Assistance of
Patients with Epilepsy**
Mladost 1, Building 65
Ent. A, App 10
1784 Sofia
Bulgaria
+359 2 740946
FAX: +359 2 740946

· CAMEROON

**Association Camerounese Contre
l'Epilepsie**
Mission Catholique Nyamanga II
B.P. 47 Ombessa

Cameroon
desimone.france@yahoo.fr

· CANADA

Epilepsy Canada
National Executive Director
1470 Peel Street, Suite 745
Montreal, Quebec H3A 1T1
Canada
+1 514 845 7855
FAX: +1 514 845 7866
crepin@epilepsy.ca
www.epilepsy.ca

· CHILE

Liga Chilena contra la Epilepsia
Patriotas Uruguayos 2236
Codigo Postal: 6501205
Santiago
Chile
+56 2699 2288
FAX: + 56 2699 4084
liche@ligaepilepsia.cl
www.ligaepilepsia.cl

· CHINA

**China Association against
Epilepsy**
3-2-703
#31 Cheng-shou-si Lu
Beijing 100078
China
+86 1390 110 2325
FAX: +8610 8762 8199
shichuoli@yahoo.com

· COLOMBIA

**Junta National Liga Colombiana
contra la Epilepsia**
Cap de Bolivar
Barrio Ternera
Calle 1a, El Eden, Y 5007 Cartagena
Colombia
+5756 618 127
FAX: +57 566 18 111
fandino@cartagena.cetcol.net.co

· CONGO

Association Fallone
188 Avenue de L'independence
Tie-Tie
BP 1533
Pointe Noire
Congo
+242 53 7134
FAX: +242 24 2958
mkounkou@yahoo.fr

· CROATIA

Croatian Association for Epilepsy
General Hospital "Sveti Duh"
Sveti Duh 64
10 000 Zagreb
Croatia
+385 1 3712143
FAX: +385 1 3712372
ivan.bielen@zg.htnet.hr

· CUBA

Capitulo Cubano de la IBE
Hospital Psiquiatrico de la Habana
Ave Independencia No 26520
Reparto Mazorra, Boyeros, Ciudad de
la Habana, CP 19220
Cuba
+537 81 1057
FAX: +537 45 1512
sglezpal@infomed.sld.cu

· CYPRUS

**Cyprus Association of Support for
People with Epilepsy**
Omirou Avenue 20, 1st Floor
PO Box 22485
1097 Nicosia
Cyprus
+357 9967 1844, +357 2266 530
FAX: +357 2251 8406
masrcodu@logos.cy.net

· CZECH REPUBLIC

Spolecnost "E"
Liskova 3
14200
Praha 4
Czech Republic
+4202 417221 36
FAX: +4202 417221 36
CEA@volny.cz
www.epilepsie.ecn.cz

- DENMARK

Dansk Epilepsiforening
Kongensgade 68, 2. Tv.
DK-5000 Odense C
Denmark
+45 6611 9091
FAX: +45 66 117 177
epilepsi@epilepsiforeningen.dk
www.epilepsiforeningen.dk

- ECUADOR

Centro Nacional de Epilepsia
APNE
Berrutieta sn y Acevedo
(Sector La Gasca)
Quito, Ecuador
+593 2 2905 405
gpesantez@uio.telconet.net

- EGYPT

Egyptian Epilepsy Association
40 Safeya Zaghlol Street
Alexandria 21111
Egypt
+203 303 3338
FAX: +203 304 7117
hhosny@internetegypt.com

- ESTONIA

Estonian Epilepsy Association
Puusepp St 2
51014 Tartu
Estonia

+372 7318515
FAX: +372 7318 509
epilepsialiit@hot.ee

- ETHIOPIA

Epilepsy Support Association of
Ethiopia (ESAE)
CEO
PO Box 25516
Code 1000.Addis Ababa
Ethiopia
+251 155 3617
FAX: +251 155 1981
zdamtie@hotmail.com

- FINLAND

Epilepsialiitto
Malmin Kauppatie 26
FIN-00700
Helsinki
Finland
+358 9350 82320
FAX: +358 9350 82322
epilepsialiitto@epilepsia.fi
www.epilepsia.fi

- FRANCE

AISPACE
38 rue du Plat
F-59000 Lille
France
+ 33 320 57 19 41
FAX: +33 320 094 124
lille.aispace@wanadoo.fr
www.epilepsies-epileptiques.com

· GAMBIA

The Gambia Epilepsy Association
#5, Dippa Dukureh Road
London Corner
PO Box 2230 Serrekunda
Gambia
+220 9955418
FAX: +220 9922414
gambiaepilepsy@yahoo.co.uk

· GEORGIA

**Epilepsy and Environment
Association of Georgia**
Department of Neurology
Tbilisi State Medical University
Jacob Nicoladze str 6, appt 22, 380079
Tbilisi
Georgia
+995 32 233 551
FAX: +995 32 221 965
natokujava@mail.ge

· GERMANY

Deutsche Epilepsie Vereinigung
Zillestrasse 102
10585 Berlin
Germany
+49 30 342 4414
FAX: +49 30 342 4466
info@epilepsie.sh
www.epilepsie.sh

· GHANA

Ghana Epilepsy Association
c/o PO Box M230
Accra
Ghana
+233 21 665 421 ext.4420
ayisu@hotmail.com

· GREECE

**Greek National Association
Against Epilepsy**
Aghia Sophia Children's Hospital
Department of Neurology/
Neurophysiology
Athens 11527
Greece
+30 210 7705 785
FAX: +30 210 7705 785
graaepil@otenet.gr

· GUATEMALA

IBE Guatemalan Chapter
6a. Calle 2–48, Zona 1
Guatemala City
Guatemala
+5022 327 258
FAX: +5022 514 008
hstokes@infovia.com.gt

· HONG KONG

Hong Kong Epilepsy Association
G/F, Block 6
Kornhill Garden
1120 King's Road
Quarry Bay

Hong Kong
+852 2794 7006
FAX: +852 2794 7178
anchor@rehabsociety.org.hk
www.hkepilepsy.com

· ICELAND

**LAUF, The Icelandic Epilepsy
Association**
Hatuni 10b
101 Reykjavik
Iceland
+354 551 4570
FAX: +354 551 4580/+354 561 8070
lauf@vortex.is
www.lauf.is/vefur

· INDIA

Indian Epilepsy Association
Specialists Clinic
No. 37, SBI
Bangalore 560 001
India
+91 080-25588274
FAX: +91 080-25588390
ieablr@vsni.net
www.indianepilepsyassociation.org

· INDONESIA

PERPEI
Bagian Neurologi FKUI
Jl. Salemba 6
Jakarta Pusat 10430
Indonesia

+62 21 335 044
FAX: +62 21 314 9424

· IRAN

Iranian Epilepsy Association
PO Box 16315-1419
Tehran
Iran
+98 21 88463355, +98 2188469153
FAX: +98 21 88463377
info@iranepi.com
www.iranepi.com

· IRELAND

Brainwave
Irish Epilepsy Association
249 Crumlin Road
Dublin 12
Ireland
+353 1 455 7500
FAX: +353 1 455 7013
mikeglynn.brainwave@epilepsy.ie
www.epilepsy.ie

· ISRAEL

Israel Epilepsy Association
4 Avodat Yisrael St
PO Box 1958
Jerusalem 91014
Israel
+97 2500 0283
FAX: +97 2253 71044
epi_eyal@hotmail.com
www.epilepsy.org.il

· ITALY

Associazone Italiana contro l'Epilessia (AICE)
via Tommaso Marino 7
20121 Milan
Italy
+3902 809 299
FAX: +3902 809 799
assaice@iperbole.bologna.it
www.aice-epilessia.it

· JAMAICA

Jamaica Epilepsy Association
44 Portview Road
Apt #6
Box 675 Kingston 8
Jamaica
+1 876 9696717
FAX: +1 876 968 1003
eperez@anngel.com.jm

· JAPAN

Japan Epilepsy Association
5F Zenkokuzaidan Building 2-2-8
Nishiwaseda Shinjuku-ku
Tokyo 162
Japan
+81 332 025 661
FAX: +81 332 027 235
www.synapse.ne.ap/jepnet

· KENYA

Kenya Association for the Welfare of Epileptics
PO Box 60790
Nairobi
Kenya
+254 2387 0885
FAX: +254 2387 4871
kawe@wananchi.com

· KOREA

Korean Epilepsy Association/Rose Club
110–021, Room No 301
Buwon Building
175–1 Buam-dong, Chongno-ku
Seoul
Korea
+822 394 2375
FAX: +822 394 7169
RoseClub@hitel.net

· LEBANON

Association of Care of Epileptic Patients
Haret Said
Facing Osseiran Palace
Property of Abdulsatar El Assi, Saida
Lebanon
+961 3388 713
FAX: +961 7731 383
epilepsyl@hotmail.com

· LITHUANIA

Lithuanian Society of Epileptic
Patients and Their Sponsors
Kaunas Medical University Hospital
Department of Neurosurgery
Eiveniu 2, LT-3007 Kaunas
Lithuania
+370 7 73 3478
FAX: +370 7 33 0477

· MALAYSIA

Persatuan Epilepsi Malaysia
Department of Neurology
Kuala Lumpur Hospital
Jalan Pahang 50586
Kuala Lumpur
Malaysia

· MALTA

Caritas Malta Epilepsy
Association
c/o Dr Janet Mifsud
5l, Gostna Triq il-Hemel
Swieqi STJ 04
Malta
+356 21 436 442
Mobile: +356 99252908
FAX: +356 320 281
www.caritasmalta.org

· MAURITIUS

EDYCS Epilepsy Group
8 Impasse Labourdonnais
Port Louis
Mauritius

edycs.org@intnet.mu
www.edycsepilepsy.intnet.mu

· MEXICO

Group "Acceptation" of Epileptics
Amsterdam 1928 No 19
Colonia Olimpica-Pedregal
Mexico 04710 DF
Mexico
FAX: +525 575 3250
www.epilepsiahoy.com

· MONGOLIA

Mongolian Epilepsy Society
NMUM, Sukhbataar distr.,
Jamyangarav str
Ulaanbaatar
Mongolia
+976 991 77 153
FAX: +976 991 132 6699
tovuudorj@yahoo.com

· MOROCCO

Association Marocaine Contre
l'Epilepsie
Neurology Department
El Razi Hospital
BP 7010 Sidi Abbad 40 000
Marrakech
Morocco
+212 6128 1437
FAX: +212 4443 2887
epilepsieassociation@yahoo.com

· NETHERLANDS

EVN
Postbus 8105
6710 AC Ede
Netherlands
+31 318 672 772
FAX: +31 318 672 770
info@epilepsievereniging.nl
www.epilepsievereniging.nl

· NEW ZEALAND

Epilepsy New Zealand (ENZ)
National Office
PO Box 1074
Hamilton
New Zealand
+64 7834 3556
FAX: +64 7834 3553
ceo@epilepsy.org.nz
www.epilepsy.org.nz

· NIGER

LNCEMNMC
Service de Psychiatrie
Hopital National de Niamey
BP 238 Niamey
Niger
+227 723392
FAX: +227 733446
ddouma@caramail.com

· NIGERIA

Epilepsy Association of Nigeria
No 2 Weeks Road by 84 Asa Road
Aba
Abia State
Nigeria
+803 433 2275
drmohaniclinic@yahoo.com

· NORWAY

Norsk Epilepsiforbund
Storgt. 39
0182 Oslo
Norway
+47 2335 3100
FAX: +47 2335 3101
nef@epilepsi.no
www.epilepsi.no

· PAKISTAN

FLAME
83 Shah Jamal Colony
Lahore
Pakistan
+9242-7581724
FAX: +9242-7572488
pprc@wol.net.pk

· PERU

Peruvian Association of Epilepsy
Jr Castilla 678
E-101
Lima 32
Peru
+51 1 460 7502
julioej@starmedia.com

· PHILIPPINES

Epilepsy Awareness and Advocacy, Inc.
17th Floor, Pacific Star Building
Sen Gil Puyat corner Makati Ave
Makati City
Philippines
+632 811 5804
FAX: +632 811 5715
guerrero.mm@uob.com.ph

· POLAND

Polish Association of People Suffering from Epilepsy
ul Fabryczna 57
15-482 Bialystok
Poland
+48 85 675 4420
FAX: +48 85 675 4420
www.padaczka.bialystok.org.pl

· PORTUGAL

Portuguese League Against Epilepsy
Av Da Boavista, 1015-6o-Sala 601
4100-428 Oporto
Portugal
+351 22 605 49 59
FAX: +351 22 605 49 59
epicentroporto@oninet.pt
www.lpce.pt

· ROMANIA

Asociatia Nationala a Bolnavilor de Epilepsie
Cluj-Napoca
Str Rene Descartes 6
Cod 400486
Romania
+4 0264 599 500, +4 0740 252 132
FAX: +4 0264 599 500
anber@epilepsie.ro
www.epilepsie.ro

· SAUDI ARABIA

Epilepsy Support and Information Centre
PO Box 3354
MBC 76
Riyadh, 11211
Saudi Arabia
+966 1 464-7272 Ext: 32833
FAX: +966 1 442 4755
contact@epilepsyinarabic.com
www.epilepsyinarabic.com

· SCOTLAND

Epilepsy Scotland
Chief Executive
48 Govan Road
Glasgow G51 1JL
Scotland
+44 141 427 4911/0808 8002200
FAX: +44 141 419 1709
enquiries@epilepsyscotland.org.uk
www.epilepsyscotland.org.uk

· SENEGAL

**Ligue Senegalaise contre
l'Epilepsie**
Clinique Neurologique
Centre Hospitalo–Universitaire
de Fann
BP 5035, Dakar-Fann
Senegal
+221 825 3678
FAX: +221 825 9227
neurofan@telecomplus.sn

· SERBIA

**Serbian-Montenegrin Society
for Epilepsy**
Slobodana Penezica-Krcuna 23
11 000 Beograd
Serbia
+381 11 686 155 ext.137
FAX: +381 11 686 656
Yusepi@ztp.co.yu

· SIERRA LEONE

**Epilepsy Association of
Sierra Leone**
10a Rokupa Estate
PO Box 381
Freetown
Sierra Leone
epilepsy-easl@yahoo.com

· SINGAPORE

**The Singapore Epilepsy
Foundation**
149 Rochor Rd
Fu Lu Shou Complex
#04-07 Singapore 188425
Singapore
+65 6334 4302
FAX: +65 6334 4669
info@epilepsy.com.sg
www.epilepsy.com.sg

· SLOVAKIA

AURA
Dubravska cesta 1
PO Box 116
84005 Bratislava 45
Slovakia
+421 915 503 193
epilepsia@pobox.sk
www.epilepsia-sk.sk

· SLOVENIA

**Slovenian League Against
Epilepsy**
Ulica Stare pravde
21000 Ljubljana
Slovenia
+386 1 432 9393 (Thursdays 4-7 pm)
FAX: + 386 1 522 9357
ljubica.vrba@kclj.si

• SOUTH AFRICA

Epilepsy South Africa
National Office
PO Box 73
Observatory 7935
Capetown
South Africa
+27 214 473 014
FAX: +27 214 485 053
info@epilepsy.org.za
www.epilepsy.org.za

• SPAIN

Asociacion Espanola de Ayuda al Epileptico
c/Berlin, 5, 40 Piso
28028 Madrid
Spain
+34 91 726 2727
FAX: +34 91 356 0926
mcdo@anit.es

• SRI LANKA

Epilepsy Association of Sri Lanka
48/93 Epitamulla road
Pitakotte
Kotte
Sri Lanka
sabrinar@sltnet.lk

• SWAZILAND

Swaziland Epilepsy Association
PO Box 5638
H100
Mbabane
Swaziland
+9268 6037032
FAX: +9268 5054727
mbusei@yahoo.com

• SWEDEN

Swedish Epilepsy Association
Executive Director
PO Box 1386
172 27 Sundbyberg
Sweden
+46 866 94106
FAX: +46 866 91588
Susanne.lund@epilepsi.se
www.epilepsi.se

• SWITZERLAND

Epi-Suisse
Seefeldstrasse 84
Postfach 313
CH-8034 Zurich
Switzerland
+41 43 488 6880
FAX: +41 43 488 6881
info@epi-suisse.ch
www.epi-suisse.ch

• TAIWAN

Taiwan Epilepsy Association
1st Floor, No 5, Alley 2, Lane 199
Tun-Hwa N. Road
Taipei 105
Taiwan
+866 225 149682
FAX: +866 225 149687
twn-tea@ms1.seeder.net
www.epilepsyorg.org.tw

· TANZANIA

**Parents Organisation for
Children with Epilepsy-POCET**
PO Box 65293
Dar Es Salaam
United Republic of Tanzania
+744 822 517
skaaya@muchs.ac.tz

· THAILAND

Epilepsy Association of Thailand
Dept of Paediatrics, Faculty of
Medicine
Ramathibodi Hospital, Mahidol
University
Rama VI Road
Bangkok 10400
Thailand
+622 201 1488
FAX: +622 201 1850
rapvs@mahidol.ac.th

· TUNISIA

Tunisian Epilepsy Association
Neurological Department
EPS Charles Nicolle
Tunis 1006
Tunisia
+216 1562 834
FAX: +216 1562 777
amel.mrabet@rns.tn

· TURKEY

**Association of Epilepsy
and Society**
Feneryolu Sokak
Kale Apartmany
5/13 Kuyubaby, 34724
Kadykoy, Istanbul
Turkey
+90 216 337 0706
FAX: +90 216 337 0676
epilepsi@gmail.com
www.epilepsi.org.tr

· UGANDA

Epilepsy Support Association
PO Box 16260
Wandegeya
Kampala
Uganda
+256 485 205 96
FAX: +256 485 205 96
amugarura@yahoo.co.uk

· UNITED KINGDOM

Epilepsy Action
New Anstey House
Gate Way Drive
Yeadon, Leeds LS19 7XY
United Kingdom
+44 113 210 8800
FAX: +44 113 391 0300
epilepsy@epilepsy.org.uk
www.epilepsy.org.uk

· URUGUAY

AUCLE
Ciudadela 1217
Montevideo
CP 11 200
Uruguay
+598 2915 9625
FAX: +598 2487 4582
abogacz@hotmail.com

· UNITED STATES

Epilepsy Foundation
4351 Garden City Drive, 5th Floor
Landover, Maryland 20785
USA
+1 301 459 3700
FAX: +1 301 459 0340
ehargis@efa.org
www.epilepsyfoundation.org

· VENEZUALA

Venezuala Bureau Nacional
Edificio Integral
Avenida Venezuela
Ubanizacion "El Rosal," Piso 1
Caracas
Venezuala
+58 414 126 6828
FAX: +58 212 951 7258
livece@lycos.com

· ZAMBIA

Epilepsy Association of Zambia
Motaxis Building
PO Box 32443 Lusaka
Zambia
+260 96 459 688
eazepilepsy01@yahoo.co.uk

· ZIMBABWE

Epilepsy Support Foundation
PO Box 104, Avondale
Old General Hospital
Mazoe Street
Harare
Zimbabwe
+263 472 4071
www.nascoh.org/members/epilepsy

Internet Resources

Note: Websites for comprehensive epilepsy centers are listed in Appendix D.

1. **American Academy of Neurology**—The Brain Matters: www.thebrainmatters.org
2. **Cyberonics** (vagus nerve stimulator)—www.cyberonics.com
3. **Clinical Trials**—www.clinicaltrials.gov, www.centerwatch.com
4. **Epilepsy Advocate**—www.epilepsyadvocate.com
5. **Epilepsy Foundation**—www.efa.org
6. **Epilepsy Information Service**— www1.wfubmc.edu/neuro/Diseases+and+Conditions/EIS.htm
7. **Epilepsy Therapy Development Project**—www.epilepsy.com
8. **Job Accommodation Network**—www.jan.wvu.edu
9. **KetoCal**—www.shsna.com/pages/ketocal.htm
10. **Seizure Dogs**—www.inch.com/~dogs/service.html, www.canineassistants.org/, ca.geocities.com/epilepsy911/seizuredogs.html
11. **National Institutes of Health, Women's Health Initiative**—www.healthtouch.com
12. **Patient Assistance Programs**—www.needymeds.com, www.rxhope.com, www.access2wellness.com
13. **Whole Brain Atlas**—www.med.harvard.edu/AANLIB/home.html
14. **Andrew Wilner, MD**—www.drwilner.org

International Internet Resources

1. **Epilepsy Action (British Epilepsy Association)**—www.epilepsy.org.uk
2. **Epilepsy Action Scotland**—www.epilepsyscotland.org.uk
3. **Epilepsy Associations of Australia**—www.epilepsy.org.au
4. **The National Society for Epilepsy (United Kingdom)**—www.epilepsynse.org.uk
5. **Epilepsy Canada**—www.epilepsy.ca
6. **National Center for Young People with Epilepsy (United Kingdom)**— www.ncype.org.uk
7. **Irish Epilepsy Association (Brainwave)**—www.epilepsy.ie/Ease/servlet/DynamicPageBuild; jsessionid=zytggc20c1?siteID=1909&categoryID=62
8. **International Bureau for Epilepsy**—www.ibe-epilepsy.org
9. **International League Against Epilepsy**—www.ilae.org
10. **Singapore Epilepsy Foundation**—www.epilepsy.com.sg
11. **Taiwan Epilepsy Society**—www.epilepsy.org.tw/ContentAspx/index.aspx

Home Safety Checklist

✓ Take precautions against burns! Cook with an electric stove (avoid gas) or microwave oven.

✓ Use rear burners when cooking.

✓ Use oven mitts.

✓ Use cart for hot food to wheel to table from stove.

✓ Install heat control devices in kitchen faucet and bathroom to prevent scalding.

✓ Carpet all floors.

✓ Use plastic containers rather than glass.

✓ Do not lock bathroom door.

✓ Take bath with only a few inches of water.

✓ Use hand-held shower head and sit during shower.

✓ Live in a one floor dwelling if possible; limit stairs.

✓ Use an iron that shuts off automatically.

✓ Avoid using a curling iron.

✓ Keep a protective screen in front of the fireplace.

✓ Avoid exposed heaters.

✓ Do not smoke cigarettes.

✓ Install smoke alarms.

✓ Check in with a friend or family member at least once a day.

✓ Keep your doctor's number by the telephone.

✓   Make sure a friend or family member has your doctor's number.

✓   Instruct friends and family on proper first aid for seizures and when to call an ambulance (Appendix J).

✓   Consider home security system with "panic button".

First Aid for Seizures

Generalized Tonic Clonic Seizure (Convulsion)

- Remain calm.
- Keep the patient from hurting himself/herself. Remove furniture and sharp objects from the area. Put something soft, such as a pillow or folded clothing under the patient's head.
- Turn the patient on his/her side to prevent choking.
- Do **NOT** put anything in the patient's mouth.
- Do not restrain the patient's movements.
- Do not attempt cardiopulmonary resuscitation (CPR) unless the patient is not breathing.
- Time the seizure. Call for emergency services (911) if jerking movements last longer than two minutes.
- After the seizure, stay with the patient until he/she is no longer confused. Check for injuries such as bruises, broken bones, cuts or head injury. Call 911 if there are serious injuries.
- Call 911 if the patient stays confused for longer than 15 minutes.
- Notify the patient's physician of the seizure.
- Do not allow the patient to drive.
- Tell the patient what happened. Ask what he/she wants to do.

Partial Complex Seizure

- Do not restrain the patient.
- Keep the patient from wandering by gently guiding him/her into a safe area.
- Do not try to reason with the patient during the seizure.
- Stay with the patient until his/her confusion clears.
- Notify the patient's physician of the seizure.
- Do not allow the patient to drive.
- Tell the patient what happened. Ask what he/she wants to do.

Note: If this is a first seizure, call 911 or bring the person to the emergency room immediately for an evaluation to find the cause of the seizure and possible treatment with antiepileptic medication.

Other Resources

**Association for the Care of
Children's Health**
3615 Wisconsin Avenue
Washington, DC 20016
(202) 244–1801

**Association for Children and
Adults with Learning Disabilities**
4156 Library Road
Pittsburgh, PA 15234
(412) 341–1515

Association for Retarded Citizens
2501 Avenue J
Arlington, TX 76011
(871) 640–0204

Children's Defense Fund
25 E Street, N.W.
Washington, DC 20001
(202) 628–8787

Council for Exceptional Children
1920 Association Drive
Reston, VA 22091–1589
(703) 620–3660

**Epilepsy Concern International
Service Group**
Executive Director
1282 Wynnewood Drive
West Palm Beach, FL 33417
(407) 683–0044

Epilepsy Information Service
Medical Center Boulevard
Winston-Salem, NC 27157–1078
(800) 642–0500

**Equal Employment Opportunity
Commission (EEOC)**
1801 L Street, N.W.
Washington, DC 20507
(800) 669–3362

Joseph P. Kennedy Foundation
1350 New York Avenue, N.W.,
Suite 500
Washington, DC 20005
(202) 393–1250

Kids on the Block
9385 C. Gerwig Lane
Columbia, MD 21046
(301) 368–5437

Medic Alert Foundation US
2323 Colorado
Turlock, CA 95382
(800) 432–5378

**National Association of
Epilepsy Centers**
5775 Wayzata Boulevard
Minneapolis, MN 55416
(952) 525–4526

**National Foundation for
Brain Research**
Suite 300
1250 24th Street N.W.
Washington, DC 20037
(202) 293–5453

National Head Injury Foundation
1776 Massachusetts Avenue
N.W., #100
Washington, DC 20036–1904
(800) 444–6443

**National Information Center
for Children and Youth with
Disabilities**
Box 1492
Washington, DC 20013–1492
(800) 695–0285

**National Institute of Neurological
Disorders and Stroke**
Office of Scientific and Health Reports
Box 5801
Bethesda, MD 20892
(800) 352–9424

**National Tuberous Sclerosis
Association, Inc.**
8181 Professional Place, Suite 110
Landover, Maryland 20785–2226
(800) 225–6872

**Office on the Americans with
Disabilities Act**
Civil Rights Division
US Department of Justice
Box 66118
Washington, DC 20035–6118
(202) 514–0301

**Resources for Children with
Special Skills**
200 Park Avenue South, Suite 816
New York, NY 10003
(212) 677–4650

Sibling Information Center
Department of Educational
Psychology
Box U-64
The University of Connecticut
Storrs, CT 06268
(203) 486–4031

Siblings for Significant Change
823 United Nations Plaza, Room 808
New York, NY 10017
(212) 420–0776

The Will Rogers Institute
785 Mamaroneck Avenue
White Plains, NY 10605
(914) 761–5550

**The Charlie Foundation to Help
Cure Pediatric Epilepsy**
501 10th Street
Santa Monica, California 90402
(800) 367–5386

**The Epilepsy Education and
Control Activities Database**
(for health care professionals)
Centers for Disease Control
and Prevention
National Center for Chronic Disease
Prevention and Health Promotion
Technical Information Services
Branch
4770 Buford Hwy, NE, MS–K13
Atlanta, Georgia 30341–3724
(404) 488–5080

Other International Epilepsy Resources

· AUSTRIA

Johanna Schallmeiner
4674 Altenhof/Hausruck
Hueb 18
07735/73–13

Inge Weidringer
4674 Altenhof
Hueb 14
07735/66–31–434

Gerlinde Prandstatter
4020 Linz
Europastrabe 38
0732/38–75–74

Peter Koller
4100 Ottensheim
Stifterstrabe 34
07234/41–69

Alois u. Uta Pucher
4774 St. Marienkirchen 143
07711/23–26

· AUSTRALIA

Melbourne Offices
818 Burke Road
Camberwell 3124
(03) 9813–2866

Western Region Office
41 Somerville Road
Yarraville 3013
(03) 9813–2866

Wendouree Community Centre
1097 Howitt Street
Wendouree 3355
(053) 381–277

Eaglehawk and Long Gully
Community Health Centre
Seymoure Street
Eaglehawk 3556
(054) 468–800

Illawarra Community Centre
265 Pakington Street
Newtown 3220
(052) 231–645

Morwell School Support
Centre
Harold Street
Morwell 3840
(051) 369–900

**Goulburn Valley Community
Care Centre**
162 Maude Street
Shepparton 3630
(058) 222–415

· CANADA

**Epilepsy Association,
Metro Toronto**
One St. Clair Avenue, East, Suite 500
Toronto ON M4T 2V7
(416) 964–9095

Epilepsy Ontario
P.O. Box 58515
197 Sheppard Avenue East
North York, Ontario
M2N 6R7
(905) 764–5099

Hamilton and District Chapter
92 King Street East, Suite 855
Hamilton, Ontario L8N 1A8
(905) 522–8487

Ottawa-Carleton Chapter
509-180 Metcalfe Street
Ottawa, Ontario
K2P 1P5
(613) 594–9255

· ENGLAND

**Mersey Region Epilepsy
Association**
Glaxo Neurological Centre
Norton Street
Liverpool L3 8LR
0151 298 2666
FAX: 0151 298 2333

· GERMANY

Geschaftsstelle der Deutschen
Sektion
der Internationalen Liga gegen
Epilepsie
Frau Ingrid Kersten Havekost
Herforder Str. 5–7
D-33602 Bielefeld
49 521 12 41 92

· HUNGARY

P. Rajna
Hungarian Chapter of the
International League Against
Epilepsy
P.O. Box 1
H–1261 Budapest 27

· ICELAND

**Icelandic Epilepsy Foundation
(L.A.U.F.)**
Laugarvegur 26
101 Reykjavik
P.O. Box 5182
125 Reykjavik
354–551–4570
FAX: 354–551–4580

· MALAYSIA

Malaysian Epilepsy Society
Neurology Department
Kuala Lumpur Hospital
50586 Kuala Lumpur
Malaysia
FAX: (603) 298-9845

· SINGAPORE

The Epilepsy Care Group
c/o Medical Alumni Association
2 College Road
Singapore 0316
Republic of Singapore
(Epilepsy support group)

· TAIWAN

Dr. Jing-Jane Tsai
President, Chinese Epilepsy Society
c/o Department of Neurology
National Cheng Kung University
Medical Center
138-Sheng-Li Road
Tainan 704
886 62 35 36 60

· TURKEY

Epilepsy Society of Turkey
Cigdem Ozkara, M.D.
I–7–C–27 7–8 Kisim Atakoy
34750 Istanbul
90212 55 90 815

· UNITED KINGDOM

**British Branch of the
International League Against
Epilepsy**
Dr. S. D. Shorvon
National Hospital for Nervous
Diseases
Queen Square
London WC1N 3 BG
44 494 873 991

· URUGUAY

Dr. Alejandro Scaramelli
Liga Uruguaya contra la Epilepsia
Hospital de Clinicas, Piso 2
Av. Italia s/n
11600 Montevideo
5982 471 221

"Plan of Action"
for the Workplace

Please see the form displayed on the following two pages.

PLAN OF ACTION

Created: _____   Updated: _____

Employee Information:

_____
Name

_____
Address

_____ __ / __ / __ ____-__-____
Phone Number   Date of Birth   SSN

Medical Documentation Attached?
_____ Yes _____ No

Emergency Contact Information:

_____
Contact's Name   Relationship

Home Phone Number: _____

Work Phone Number: _____

_____
Doctor/Hospital

Disability and/or Limitation(s): _____
_____

Things to watch out for (Warning Signs):
a. _____
b. _____
c. _____

Action Plan:
a. _____
b. _____
c. _____
d. _____
e. _____

Additional Comments:

_____   _____   _____   _____
Employee's Signature   Date   Employer's Signature   Date

| Created: 12/3/99 | **_PLAN OF ACTION_** | Updated: 7/11/01 |

Employee Information:

John P. Smith
Name

222 High Street Morgantown, WV 26505
Address

(304) 293-5555   06/18/68   123-45-6789
Phone Number   Date of Birth   SSN

Medical Documentation Attached?
_X_ Yes ___ No

Emergency Contact Information:

Sarah Smith _____ Wife
Contact's Name _____ Relationship

Home Phone Number: (304) 293-5555

Work Phone Number: (304) 293-1234

Dr. Robert Dell --- General Hospital
Doctor/Hospital

Disability and/or Limitation(s): Food allergy to peanuts and tree nuts

Things to watch out for (Warning Signs):
a. John will experience tingling in the mouth.
b. John's lips and mouth will swell.
c. John will have difficulty breathing and may make wheezing sounds.
d. If able, John will inject himself with epinephrine using his EpiPen®
   and will attempt to signal co-worker or supervisor. He carries the
   epinephrine with him at all times and wears a medical alert bracelet.
   Extra epinephrine is stored in his upper right desk drawer.

Action Plan:
a. Call 911; have someone stay with John while another person goes to
   meet the ambulance.
b. Assist John to a comfortable position and loosen his tie if he is
   wearing one.
c. The epinephrine may take 5 to 15 minutes to work.
d. Remain calm and reassure John that help is coming.

Additional Comments:
1. Co-Workers, Susie Johnson and David Jones, will carry radios to hear
   John's emergency signal.
2. Supervisor will call John's emergency contact person.

| _John P. Smith_ | 7/11/01 | _Lydia S. Brown_ | 7/11/01 |
| Employee's Signature | Date | Employer's Signature | Date |

The Job Accommodation Network (JAN) is a service of the U.S. DOL Office of Disability
Employment Policy. Employers are not required to use this form under the ADA or any
other employment law. JAN provides this document as a tool to help identify and implement
accommodations for people with epilepsy or other seizure activity. This document may be
reproduced and freely distributed, so long as its nature and content is not altered, and it is
properly referenced.

*This form may **NOT** be kept in an employee's personnel file. It must be kept in the
employee's medical file.*

Glossary of Acronyms

ACTH	adrenocorticotropic hormone
ADHD	attention deficit hyperactivity disorder
AED	antiepileptic drug
AES	American Epilepsy Society
AVM	arteriovenous malformation
BECRS	benign epilepsy of childhood with Rolandic spikes
CAT	computerized axial tomography
CBC	complete blood count
CBTL	carbamazepine extended release (Carbatrol®)
CBZ	carbamazepine (Tegretol®)
CCTV/EEG	closed circuit television/electroencephalography
CNS	central nervous system
CT	computerized axial tomography (same as CAT)
EEG	electroencephalograph
EF	Epilepsy Foundation
EMU	epilepsy monitoring unit
EPC	epilepsia partialis continua
FBM	felbamate
FDA	Food and Drug Administration
GBP	gabapentin (Neurontin®)
GTC	generalized tonic clonic seizure (convulsion)
IRB	institutional review board
IV	intravenous
JME	juvenile myoclonic epilepsy

LEV	levetiracetam (Keppra®)
LFTS	liver function tests
LTG	lamotrigine (Lamictal®)
MEG	magnetoencephalography
MRA	magnetic resonance angiography
MRI	magnetic resonance imaging
MRS	magnetic resonance spectroscopy
MTS	mesial temporal sclerosis
OCBZ	oxcarbazepine (Trileptal®)
PB	phenobarbital
PDR	Physicians' Desk Reference
PET	positron emission tomography
PHT	phenytoin (Dilantin®)
PI	principal investigator
PRM	primidone (Mysoline®)
SPECT	single photon emission computed tomography
TGB	tiagabine (Gabitril®)
TLE	temporal lobe epilepsy
TPM	topiramate (Topamax®)
VNS	vagus nerve stimulator
VPA	valproic acid (Depakene®)
VR	vocational rehabilitation
ZNS	zonisamide (Zonegran®)

Managed Care

DM	disease management
HMO	health maintenance organization
IPA	independent practice association
MCO	managed care organization
PHO	physician-hospital organization
PPO	preferred provider organization

Glossary of Terms

Absence seizure A type of generalized seizure usually seen in children, characterized by staring, accompanied by a 3 per second spike and wave pattern on the electroencephalograph (EEG). These seizures respond well to antiepileptic medication and most children outgrow them.

Arteriovenous malformation A tangle of arteries and veins in the brain that can cause headaches, seizures, or bleeding. Often requires surgery.

Ataxia A type of clumsiness, often the result of too much antiepileptic medication.

Aura A warning that a seizure may begin, often described as a "funny feeling." An aura is actually a small seizure that may develop into a larger seizure, or it may disappear.

Automatisms Involuntary movements that may accompany seizures, such as chewing, lip smacking, fumbling at a button, hand rubbing, or pulling on clothes.

Benign Epileptiform Transients of Sleep On the EEG, these small spikes can be unilateral or bilateral. Also known as small sharp spikes of sleep (SSS), these benign discharges should not be confused with epileptic spikes.

Benign Familial Neonatal Convulsions Occurring primarily on days 2 and 3 after birth, these clonic and apneic seizures are dominantly inherited. Only 14 percent of these infants develop epilepsy.

Benign Myoclonic Epilepsy in Infancy In this rare disorder, myoclonic seizures occur in normal children in the first or second year of life. Approximately one-third have a family history of seizures. Developmental delay often occurs. Seizures respond well to antiepileptic medication. Convulsions may occur during adolescence.

Benign Neonatal Convulsions These clonic or apneic seizures occur without known cause on day 5 after birth (fifth day fits). The electroencephalogram (EEG) may show alternating theta waves. Development is normal, and seizures do not recur.

Benign Rolandic Epilepsy Accounts for almost 25 percent of seizures appearing in children from ages 5 to 14 years. They are not always treated with antiepileptic medication because seizures are typically outgrown by adolescence.

Catamenial Epilepsy Some women have seizures only at the time of menstruation. Many other women note an increase in seizures in the perimenstrual (days −3 to 3), ovulatory (days 10 to 13), or latter half of their menstrual cycle. Studies report a wide range of 10 to 78% of women with catamenial epilepsy. These seizure patterns become evident when women carefully document seizure frequency and menstruation on a calendar. An increase in the estradiol: progesterone ratio may be responsible for the increase in seizures. Identifying a hormonal link to seizure frequency may allow for more targeted treatment.

Childhood Absence Epilepsy (Petit Mal, True Petit Mal, Pyknolepsy) Characterized by multiple staring spells, this seizure type occurs in preschool or school-aged children who otherwise are neurologically normal. Seizures may be provoked by hyperventilation. The electroencephalogram (EEG) reveals generalized 3-Hz spike and wave. Forty percent of patients also have generalized tonic-clonic seizures. Ethosuximide or valproate readily controls staring spells. Children usually outgrow this syndrome, which is a type of primary generalized epilepsy (see *Absence Seizure*).

Clonic Seizure   An epileptic seizure characterized by jerking.

Comprehensive Epilepsy Program   Often found at a medical school (Comprehensive Epilepsy Centers Directory—Appendix D), these programs combine the skills of an epileptologist, neurosurgeon, neuropsychiatrist, neuropsychologist, neuroradiologist, nurse clinician, social worker, and others in a dedicated team designed to help patients with epilepsy. A comprehensive epilepsy center can provide advanced neurodiagnostic studies such as magnetic resonance imaging (MRI), single photon emission computed tomography (SPECT), positron emission tomography (PET), and video-EEG monitoring. Investigational antiepileptic drugs (AEDs) and other research protocols may also be available. Patients likely to benefit from a comprehensive epilepsy center are those with anatomical lesions referred for epilepsy surgery, persistent seizures despite treatment with multiple AEDs, or suspected nonepileptic seizures.

Computerized Axial Tomography   A CAT or CT scan. This type of x-ray uses a computer to assemble multiple images, producing a detailed picture of the skull and brain.

Convulsion   A seizure characterized by stiffening of the body and jerking, excess salivation (foaming at the mouth), and loss of control of urine, followed by a period of confusion. Also called a generalized tonic clonic or grand mal seizure.

Corpus Callosum   The white matter that connects the two hemispheres of the brain. A corpus callosotomy is an operation in which a part or all of this structure is cut, disconnecting the two hemispheres. This surgery is typically reserved for patients with intractable generalized epilepsy, such as the Lennox-Gastaut syndrome.

Cortical Dysplasia   Broad category of neuronal migration disorders. Examples include agyria, laminar heterotopia, microdysgenesis, pachygyria, and polymicrogyria. These developmental abnormalities often lead to childhood epilepsy.

Cytochrome P450 An enzyme system consisting of a number of isoenzymes responsible for the metabolism, primarily in the liver, of many antiepileptic drugs (AEDs). For example, cytochrome P450 3A4 metabolizes carbamazepine, whereas phenytoin is metabolized by cytochrome P450 2C9. Other cytochrome enzymes participate in the metabolism of these drugs as well. Cytochrome P450 activity may be induced or inhibited by AEDs and many other drugs, affecting the rate of AED metabolism and resultant serum AED levels. The potential effect on the cytochrome P450 system should be assessed whenever a new drug is added to (or removed from) a patient's regimen.

Déjà Vu A sensation that a new experience has occurred before. Déjà vu is a disturbance of higher cerebral function characteristically due to a partial seizure localized in the temporal lobe. A déjà vu sensation may occur as an aura prior to a complex partial or generalized seizure.

Depth Electrodes Invasive electrodes used to determine the seizure focus when scalp electroencephalograms (EEGs) remain inconclusive. Typically, four to six electrodes are placed stereotactically into the brain under computed axial tomography (CAT) or magnetic resonance imaging (MRI) guidance through small holes drilled into the skull. These electrodes are associated with a small risk of hemorrhage and infection.

DigiTrace An ambulatory electroencephalogram (EEG) monitoring system that uses digital technology. The patient has EEG electrodes connected to the scalp and then takes the DigiTrace computer home for 1 to several days. The device contains computer software that records background samples, spikes, electrographic seizures, and push-button events. These are later downloaded and reviewed on paper or a computer screen. DigiTrace can also record video along with the EEG.

Double Blind A clinical trial in which medication is coded so that neither the doctor nor the patient knows whether placebo or active medication is being used. Double-blind studies help prevent bias.

Drop Attack Often seen in Lennox-Gastaut syndrome, a type of seizure that causes the person to suddenly fall. May cause injuries, especially of the face and head.

Electrode A small metal contact attached to a wire designed to record brain waves from the scalp or inside the brain.

Electroencephalogram Discovered by Hans Berger in 1929, the electroencephalogram (EEG) remains an essential component of all clinical neurophysiology laboratories. The pattern of human brain waves corresponds to levels of mental alertness, sleep stages, and the presence or absence of epileptic activity. Scalp electrodes distributed in an array over the head detect the brain's electricity, which is then filtered, amplified, and continuously recorded on paper by voltage-sensitive pens or displayed on a computer screen. Typically, 16 channels of electrical activity from different brain areas are recorded. A standard EEG represents 20 minutes of continuous recording. Prolonged EEGs can save hours or days of collected information to a computer hard drive. To enhance review, software can search the record for spikes and subclinical seizures.

Electrographic Seizures (Subclinical Seizures) Seizures detected on the electroencephalogram (EEG) that do not produce clinical symptoms.

Encephalitis An inflammation in the brain caused by infection. May be accompanied by seizures and result in epilepsy later in life.

Epilepsia Partialis Continua A rare seizure type that consists of repeated jerking (focal motor seizures), usually of the face or arm, which continues for hours or days. Consciousness is preserved. Postictal weakness occurs. Rasmussen's encephalitis is commonly responsible, but these enduring seizures may also be caused by Alper's disease, subacute type of delayed measles encephalitis, and mitochondrial encephalomyopathy with lactic acidosis and stroke-like episodes.

Epileptic Focus   The site in the brain where a seizure begins.

Epileptic Syndrome   A constellation of symptoms and signs, seizure types, etiology, anatomy, age of onset, precipitating factors, and other characteristics. Defining an epilepsy syndrome guides treatment and refines prognosis. Examples of epilepsy syndromes are Lennox-Gastaut, benign Rolandic epilepsy, childhood absence epilepsy, juvenile myoclonic epilepsy, and West's syndrome.

Epileptologist   A neurologist with special training who treats patients with epilepsy.

Febrile Seizure   A seizure caused by a high fever in children under the age of 5. Most of these children do not develop epilepsy.

Fit   A seizure.

Generalized Seizure   A seizure that affects both hemispheres of the brain.

Generalized Tonic Clonic Seizure   A convulsion.

Grand Mal Seizure   A convulsion.

Grid   An array of electrodes placed on the brain to locate a seizure focus or map speech.

Half-Life   The time required for half the amount of a drug to disappear from the body.

Health Management Organization   Members of this type of health plan pay a fixed monthly fee, regardless of their health care needs. They must use certain doctors and hospitals. Expensive tests and services may be more difficult to obtain.

Hemimegalencephaly   A congenital malformation where the affected side of the brain has a larger hemisphere and ventricle. The cortex is excessively thick and does not function normally.

Hemispherectomy A type of epilepsy surgery in which one of the hemispheres of the brain is removed or disconnected. Can be extremely helpful in controlling seizures in appropriate patients.

Hertz A unit of frequency (cycles per second). Brain waves are measured in hertz (Hz): for example, background alpha rhythm might occur on the electroencephalogram (EEG) at 10 cycles per second, or 10 Hz.

Hippocampal Sclerosis An abnormality in the hippocampus, a part of the brain important for memory. The hippocampus is in the temporal lobe and often associated with temporal lobe epilepsy. Hippocampal sclerosis may be identified on magnetic resonance imaging (MRI). People with epilepsy due to hippocampal sclerosis may have difficulty controlling their seizures with antiepileptic medications, but often do well with epilepsy surgery.

Hypsarrhythmia A dramatic abnormal pattern of irregular high-amplitude slow waves and spikes on the electroencephalogram (EEG) seen in West's syndrome.

Indemnity Insurance Allows purchasers to choose their own doctor. Pays a percentage of the total bill after a deductible.

Infantile Spasms A type of seizure that occurs in infants, characterized by frequent jerks of the body. Infantile spasms, hypsarrhythmia (see above), and mental retardation comprise West's syndrome.

Intractable Epilepsy Refers to seizures that cannot be stopped by trials of several appropriate antiepileptic medications. Also referred to as refractory or uncontrolled epilepsy.

Intravenous Medications or fluids administered through a needle into a vein.

Juvenile Absence Epilepsy A type of epilepsy occurring around puberty with absence seizures. Convulsions occur in half the patients.

Juvenile Myoclonic Epilepsy of Janz   This type of epilepsy begins in the teenage years and is characterized by myoclonic seizures, which occur more often when the person is fatigued. Convulsions and absence seizures may also occur. Patients rarely outgrow this epilepsy syndrome, but response to antiepileptic medication, particularly valproate, is excellent.

Ketogenic Diet   A high-fat, low-carbohydrate diet with adequate protein, the ketogenic diet is another approach to seizure control that works well in some patients. This diet must be supervised by a neurologist and dietician as serious side effects may occur.

Lennox-Gastaut Syndrome   A type of epilepsy beginning in early childhood characterized by frequent seizures and multiple seizure types. These children have mental retardation and slow spike and wave complexes on their electroencephalograms (EEGs). This type of epilepsy is extremely difficult to control.

Liver Function Test Abnormality   An elevation of liver enzymes, which may result from antiepileptic drugs and many other causes. This is a common finding on blood tests and not a cause for concern unless the level is very high.

Low White Count   An abnormality detected on a complete blood count (CBC), which may be a side effect of antiepileptic medication.

Magnetic Resonance Angiography   A magnetic resonance imaging scan of the blood vessels of the brain. Does not require any contrast material (dye).

Magnetic Resonance Imaging   A scan that uses a powerful magnet instead of x-rays to form an extremely detailed image of the brain.

Magnetic Resonance Spectroscopy   A new method of measuring brain metabolism using a magnetic resonance imaging scanner.

Magnetoencephalography   An experimental device that measures minute magnetic fields produced by ionic currents in the brain.

Magnetoencephalography complements electroencephalography (EEG) and may help localize an epileptic focus.

Medicaid A state-administered program of federal financial assistance primarily for families with children, the aged, blind, and disabled.

Medicare A federally funded health insurance program primarily for people age 65 and older and the disabled.

Meningitis An inflammation of the coverings of the brain.

Mental Retardation Decreased intellectual functioning with a very low IQ (<70), affecting language, motor, social, and visual abilities. One-third of patients with severe mental retardation requiring institutionalization also have epilepsy.

Monotherapy Single antiepileptic drug treatment for epilepsy. Compared to polytherapy (more than one drug), the advantages of monotherapy include absence of drug-drug interactions, fewer side effects, lower cost, and simpler dosing.

Myoclonus Brief motor jerks that may represent epileptic seizures. May be seen in a number of different epilepsy syndromes, such as myoclonic epilepsy of Janz.

Neuron A nerve cell. Billions of neurons interact to make up a working brain. Epileptic discharges are produced when groups of neurons misfire.

Neuronal Migration Disorders Brain malformations that may cause epilepsy.

Nonconvulsive Status Epilepticus A prolonged seizure state characterized by confusion, mental slowness, stupor, or coma. Nonconvulsive status epilepticus may be due to either persistent absence seizures or partial complex seizures. An electroencephalogram (EEG) is needed to confirm this diagnosis.

Nonepileptic Seizures   Clinically resemble epileptic seizures but without epileptic discharges from the brain. Also called psychogenic or nonepileptic seizures, most often caused by severe psychosocial stress. Sometimes physiological events such as syncope, tics, or transient ischemic attacks are also mistaken for epileptic seizures. The diagnosis of unexplained spells may be very difficult to make with only the patient as witness. Consequently, video/EEG may be necessary.

Nystagmus   Bouncing eye movements, often the result of antiepileptic medication toxicity.

Open Label   A clinical trial in which the name and dosage of the investigational drug are known to the investigator and patient.

Partial Complex Seizure   A seizure that begins in a specific location in the brain and alters consciousness, causing confusion. Temporal lobe partial complex seizures are sometimes called psychomotor seizures. Typically, these last from 30 seconds to several minutes. Automatisms, such as chewing, fumbling with clothes, lip smacking, and swallowing commonly occur. Because of the alteration in consciousness, patients may not always be aware that they had a seizure. Partial complex seizures may be self-limited or evolve into secondarily generalized seizures.

Partial Seizure   A seizure that begins in a specific location in the brain, such as the temporal lobe. Partial seizures are the most common seizure type in adults. Partial seizures are categorized as either "simple" or "complex" (see below).

Partial Simple Seizure   A seizure that begins in a specific location in the brain but does not alter consciousness. It may produce an abnormal sensation, such as an unpleasant smell or a motor movement. An epileptic aura is also a partial simple seizure. Partial simple seizures may be self-limited or evolve into partial complex or secondarily generalized seizures.

Petit Mal Seizure   Same as absence seizure.

Pharmacokinetic Interactions   An antiepileptic drug may sometimes interact with another drug, raising or lowering its serum level. For example, valproate may increase the levels of lamotrigine. A thorough knowledge of pharmacokinetic interactions is necessary when prescribing polytherapy. Pharmacokinetic interactions may be assessed by measuring antiepileptic drug levels.

Placebo   An inactive substance sometimes used as a basis for comparison when new drugs are tested.

Polycystic Ovary Syndrome   Hormonal and metabolic abnormalities and polycystic ovaries that appear to be increased in women with epilepsy. Valproate may be responsible for polycystic ovary syndrome in some women.

Polytherapy   Treatment with multiple drugs. For some patients, seizure control cannot be achieved with one antiepileptic drug (monotherapy).

Positron Emission Tomography   A scan that uses an injection of radioactive tracer to measure brain metabolism in an effort to locate the seizure focus. Often part of the evaluation before seizure surgery.

Postictal   The period immediately after a seizure.

Preferred Provider Organization   An insurance plan that allows members to use specified doctors in a discounted fee for service arrangement.

Prolactin   A hormone that increases after an epileptic seizure. Prolactin levels may be useful in the diagnosis of nonepileptic seizures.

Protocol   The specific manner in which a clinical trial is conducted. When all the sites of a clinical trial use the same protocol, the results can be pooled for analysis.

Pseudoseizures   See *nonepileptic seizures.*

Rasmussen's Encephalitis   Progressive brain inflammation that produces uncontrolled seizures. May be successfully treated by hemispherectomy.

Single Photon Emission Computerized Tomography   A scan that uses an injection of a radioactive tracer to measure blood flow in the brain. Typically two SPECT scans are done, one during a seizure and one in between seizures. SPECT scans can help identify a seizure focus in preparation for seizure surgery.

Spike   A characteristic finding on the electroencephalograph (EEG) in patients with epilepsy. A spike is the result of an abnormal synchronized electrical discharge in a population of neurons.

Status Epilepticus   A condition of recurrent seizures on the same day or prolonged seizures requiring immediate medical attention. Status epilepticus can be life threatening.

Subclinical Seizures   See *electrographic seizures.*

Subdural Electrodes   Small metal contacts placed on the cerebral cortex to record electrical activity. Subdural electrodes can help find the seizure focus in preparation for epilepsy surgery. They may also be used for other types of brain mapping.

Sudden Unexpected (Unexplained) Death in Epilepsy (SUDEP)   Sudden unexpected death in epilepsy is a rare cause of death for people with epilepsy. There is no known cause.

Telemetry   Continuous monitoring of the electroencephalogram (EEG), often with video.

Temporal Lobe   A part of the brain important in memory and speech. Often the site of the epileptic focus.

Temporal Lobectomy   An operation to remove the left or right temporal lobe, whichever one is responsible for the seizures. People with temporal lobe epilepsy often are cured of disabling seizures after a temporal lobectomy.

Therapeutic Range A guide, and only a guide, for antiepileptic drug levels. For example, the therapeutic range of phenytoin is 10 to 20 µg/mL. Patients often require more or less antiepileptic medication to control their seizures than suggested by the therapeutic range listed on the laboratory report.

Todd's Paralysis A temporary weakness of an arm, leg, or other body part after a seizure.

Tonic seizure An epileptic seizure characterized by stiffening.

Toxicity An undesirable effect of medication such as drowsiness, dizziness, difficulty concentrating, or trouble walking.

Tuberous Sclerosis An inherited disorder, typically with abnormalities of the brain, skin, and other organs, mental retardation, and seizures. Tuberous sclerosis accounts for 25% of cases of infantile spasms.

Vagus Nerve Stimulator A device designed to control seizures, similar to a cardiac pacemaker, but with an electrode attached to the vagus nerve in the neck. Many patients using the vagus nerve stimulator experience a decrease in seizure frequency.

Wada Test Named after its developer, Dr. Juhn Wada, this is an injection into the carotid artery of amobarbital (Amytal). It is used to determine the location of the brain's speech center and test memory prior to epilepsy surgery.

West's Syndrome A type of epilepsy in infants characterized by abrupt spasms of the body that usually occur in clusters (infantile spasms), mental retardation, and an abnormal pattern on the electroencephalograph (EEG) called hypsarrhythmia.

Bibliography

Information Books for People with Epilepsy

Complementary and Alternative Therapies for Epilepsy, Orrin Devinsky, Steven C. Schachter, Steven Pacia (eds.), Demos Medical Publishing, New York, 2005.

Epilepsy: Patient and Family Guide, 3rd Edition, Orrin Devinsky, Demos Health, New York, 2008.

Epilepsy and Pregnancy, Stacey Chillemi and Blanca Vazquez, Demos Medical Publishing, New York, 2006.

Epilepsy: A New Approach, Adrienne Richard and Joel Reiter, Walker and Company, New York, 1995.

Epilepsy: A Guide to Balancing Your Life: American Academy of Neurology Press Quality of Life Guide, Ilo E. Leppik, Demos Medical Publishing, New York, 2007.

Epilepsy A to Z: A Glossary of Epilepsy Terminology, Peter W. Kaplan, Pierre Loiseau, Robert S. Fisher, Pierre Jallon, Demos Medical Publishing, New York, 1995.

Growing Up with Epilepsy: A Practical Guide for Parents, Lynn Bennett Blackburn, Demos Medical Publishing, 2003.

Health Insurance Resources: A Guide for People with Chronic Disease and Disability, 2nd Edition, Dorothy E. Northrop, Stephen Cooper, Kimberly Calder, Demos Medical Publishing, 2007.

Insurance Solutions: Plan Well, Live Better, Laura D. Cooper, Demos Medical Publishing, New York, 2002.

Living Well with Epilepsy and other Seizure Disorders, Carl W. Bazil, Harper-Collins Publishers, Inc., New York, 2004.

Living Well with Epilepsy, 2nd Edition, Robert J. Gumnit, Demos Medical Publishing, New York, 1996.

The Amazing Brain, Robert Ornstein, Richard F. Thompson, illustrated by David Macaulay, Houghton Mifflin Company, Boston, 1984.

The Ketogenic Diet: A Treatment for Children and Others with Epilepsy, 4th Edition, John M. Freeman, Eric H. Kossoff, Jennifer B. Freeman, Millicent T. Kelly, Demos Medical Publishing, New York, 2006.

Keto Kid: Helping Your Child Succeed on the Ketogenic Diet, Deborah Snyder, Demos Medical Publishing, New York, 2007.

Seizures and Epilepsy in Childhood: A Guide for Parents, John M. Freeman, Eileen P. G. Vining, Diana J. Pillas, The Johns Hopkins University Press, Baltimore, 1991.

The Falling Sickness: A History of Epilepsy from the Greeks to the Beginnings of Modern Neurology, Oswei Temkin, The Johns Hopkins University Press, Baltimore, 1994.

Books Written By and/or About People With Epilepsy

A Bomb in the Brain: A Heroic Tale of Science, Surgery, and Survival, Steve Fishman, Avon Books, New York, 1988.

Embrace the Dawn: One Woman's Story of Triumph Over Epilepsy, Andrea Davidson, Sylvan Creek Press, McCall, 1989.

Epilepsy, I Can Live With That! Writings by People with Epilepsy, Sue Goss (ed.), Epilepsy Foundation of Victoria, Inc., Victoria, Australia, 1995.

Equal Partners, A Physician's Call for a New Spirit of Medicine, Jody Heymann, Little, Brown and Company, Boston, 1995.

Miles to Go Before I Sleep, My Grateful Journey Back from the Hijacking of Egypt Air Flight 648, Jackie Nink Pflug, Hazelden Foundation, Center City, Minnesota, 1996.

Mom, I Have a Staring Problem*, Marian and Tiffany Buckel, Marian Buckel, Bradenton, 1992.

Epilepsy in Our Words: Personal Accounts of Living with Seizures, Steven C. Schachter (ed.), Oxford University Press, Oxford, 2007.

Epilepsy in Our View: Stories From Friends and Family of People with Epilepsy, Steven C. Schachter (ed.), Oxford University Press, Oxford, 2007.

Epilepsy on Our Terms: Stories by Children with Seizures and Their Parents, Steven C. Schachter, Georgia D. Montouris, John M. Pellock (eds.), Oxford University Press, Oxford, 2007.

Epilepsy in Our Experience: Accounts of Health Care Professionals, Steven C. Schachter (ed.), Oxford University Press, Oxford, 2007.

Epilepsy in Our Lives: Women Living with Epilepsy, Steven C. Schachter (ed.), Oxford University Press, Oxford, 2007.

Epilepsy in Our World: Stories of Living with Seizures From Around the World, Steven C. Schachter (ed.), Oxford University Press, Oxford, 2007.

---

*For children

Index

241

OTHER DEMOS TITLES ON EPILEPSY FOR PATIENTS AND THEIR FAMILIES

Orrin Devinsky, *Epilepsy: Patient and Family Guide,* 3rd ed., 2008, 408 pages, $16.95, ISBN: 9781932603415.

Ilo E. Leppik, *Epilepsy: A Guide to Balancing Your Life,* 2007, 192 pages, $19.95, ISBN: 9781932603200.

Deborah Snyder, *Keto Kid: Helping Your Child Succeed on the Ketogenic Diet,* 2007, 176 pages, $16.95, ISBN: 9781932603293.

John M. Freeman, Eric H. Kossoff, Jennifer B. Freeman, and Millicent T. Kelly, *The Ketogenic Diet: A Treatment for Children and Others with Epilepsy,* 4th ed., 2007, 328 pages, $24.95, ISBN: 9781932603187.

Stacey Chillemi and Blanca Vazquez, *Epilepsy and Pregnancy,* 2006, 144 pages, $16.95, ISBN: 9781932603156.

Lynn Bennett Blackburn, *Growing Up with Epilepsy,* 2003, 168 pages, $19.95, 9781888799743.

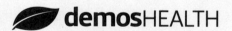 **demos**HEALTH

386 Park Avenue South, Suite 301
New York, NY 10016
Tel: 800-532-8663
Fax: 212-683-0118
orderdept@demosmedpub.com
www.demosmedpub.com